The Ghost Remover Chronicles

The Fascinating Journey of
Hypnotherapist Robert Major
Into the Spirit Realm

𝕲𝖍𝖔𝖘𝖙 𝕹𝖊𝖜𝖘 𝕾𝖔𝖚𝖗𝖈𝖊: 𝖁𝖔𝖑𝖚𝖒𝖊 𝕴
By L. Sims

ISBN: 9781091297210

DEDICATION

This book is dedicated to the seen and unseen
helpers and adepts that guide us all.
It is their selfless devotion to helping others
that has inspired me to share
this remarkable story.

CONTENTS

ACKNOWLEDGMENTS

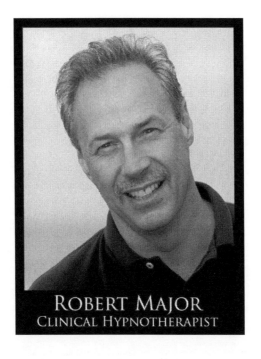

ROBERT MAJOR
CLINICAL HYPNOTHERAPIST

My sincere thanks go out to Robert Major and his Ghost Remover team for their willingness to allow me to observe and document the wide variety of situations their work entails. Without their unique and varied explorations into the spirit realm, this book would not have been possible.

I also wish to thank Editor, Jennifer Wiegand for her insightful advice and steadfast support throughout this entire project.

CHAPTER 1:
THE ROAD TO DISCOVERY

At the center of the *Attachment* and ghost removal endeavor is Hypnotherapist Robert Major. His experiences are numerous and sometimes complicated. He has the inquisitiveness and tenacity to follow the many leads he has encountered, not knowing where they would take him.

To begin, allow me to tell you about Robert Major. He was born in upstate New York where he had a tempestuous childhood chock-full of challenges. Raised by a single mother and sometimes foster care, he learned early on to figure out things for himself. He has a very charismatic personality and a wonderful sense of humor that proved to be an effective counterbalance to the instability of his youth.

Robert has an insatiable curiosity that he feeds with books, travel and new experiences. He has been all over the world learning first-hand about vastly different people, cultures and their diverse ways of looking at life, death and the afterlife. No doubt, Robert's hypnosis work is a kind of travel as well.

In his early twenties Robert asked a friend what the most

influential book he had ever read was. That friend replied *Seth Speaks*. He was intrigued at the time but had forgotten about it until one day, not long afterwards, while browsing the shelves in a used bookstore, a book fell off the shelf and bumped Robert in the shoulder. He caught the book before it hit the ground. It was *Seth Speaks*. In that book, Jane Roberts channels a spirit being by the name of Seth. The book describes the wisdom Seth has to share with us. Robert was deeply impressed as well and realized that a metaphysical path may be the first step in his quest for truth.

As a young man, he was innately inspired. He set out to overcome his fears by challenging himself to face the four elements:

Earth: He took long hikes alone in the wilderness.
Air: He went skydiving.
Fire: He did fire-walking.
Water: He overcame a fear of drowning and learned to swim.

However, it was fire-walking which proved to be the most profound and life changing experience for Robert. After days of preparation, he joined a small group of people guided by Coach and Author Anthony Robbins as each took their turn walking down a long row of hot coals. None of them were burned. This experience made him realize that reality was not as concrete as we think, but instead flexible.

Robert has many talents. He has worked as an entrepreneur and been a radio personality. He loves to cook for family and friends. But most know him as a clinical hypnotherapist. He has studied and been certified by the best in the field of hypnotherapy and stage hypnosis. They include Gil Boyne, Ormand McGill and Atilla. During his hypnosis shows, Robert gained a lot of experience hypnotizing people under adverse conditions such as with extreme distractions. Yet he found himself dissatisfied. To Robert, hypnosis had the potential to be so much more than entertainment value. Though he enjoyed making people laugh, he longed to explore the deeper ramifications of what hypnosis had to offer.

He read authors like James Van Praagh who is well versed in spirit communication and Dr. Brian Weiss known for applying hypnosis to explore past lives. However, Edgar Cayce was exceptionally influential. He was unique in that he could hypnotize himself. Referred to as self-hypnosis, during the early 1900's, Cayce gave 14,000 readings while in trance.[1] Nicknamed "The Sleeping Prophet" he answered questions on subjects as varied as healing, reincarnation, wars, Atlantis, and future events while in a trance. This helped Robert realize there was a much greater potential for his trance work.

These influences and events ignited Robert's curiosity. They led Robert to explore areas like past lives and communicating with deceased spirits. Since the time of his first experience with the spirit realm, Robert scheduled meetings twice a week at his home. For the next five years, people gathered there to explore all aspects of the spirit

---

[1] Suggested Resource: Edgar Cayce's Association for Research and Enlightenment (A.R.E.) online at edgarcayce.org.

realm. It eventually evolved into working with spirit guides to help clients who were experiencing challenges in life.

With the help and guidance from the team Robert had assembled, communications took place on a regular basis that helped both the living and the deceased. The spirit guide named Rajah was the first in the long line of many guides that have presented themselves as helpers which have resulted in the development of many skills. One is the identification and clearing of ghosts that *Attach* referred to as the Ghost Remover process.

As a result of the uncommon synchronicity of events in my life, I have followed Robert Major's hypnosis exploration for nearly twenty years now. It has afforded me the unique privilege of having witnessed the evolution of his journey from hypnotherapy to working with the spirit realm to his discovery of the *Attachment* epidemic and how to cope with it. I have also been a benefactor of his work and the Ghost Remover process with the clearing of the *Attachment* that plagued me. Originally known for his hypnotherapy, he is now known as the Ghost Remover. This is his saga.

The year was 1999 when Robert Major responded to a disturbing call from his sister, Antoinette. She phoned to say she was experiencing strange happenings in her house. She reported that objects had been moved while she was out of the room, and other incidences like this had escalated over the past few weeks. When a loaf of bread flew out of the cupboard and hit her in the face, she panicked and asked him to come right over.

Well versed in hypnosis by that time, Robert had heard about its potential to heighten one's ability to communicate with the spirit realm. So, shortly after arriving, he placed Antoinette in trance. She began communicating with the spirit who was positioned a few feet in front of the chair in which she sat. He reported to her that he had been causing all the objects to move about. They discovered he was a young boy. Remarkably, Robert and I observed Antoinette animatedly communicating with the boy who was invisible to our eyes.

Antoinette was laughing at the boy's antics. "He wants me to guess his name." She said. He's showing me a baby kangaroo. "I don't get it." Antoinette said as she raised her hands in frustration. The invisible boy spoke but only she could hear him. "Oh. His name is Joey!" she exclaimed. "A 'Joey' is a baby kangaroo!" After questioning the boy for a while they discovered that he was her half brother who had died before Antoinette was born. He explained that he felt alone where he was in the spirit realm and liked visiting Antoinette. He also enjoyed visiting another brother named Mark. Robert asked Joey what he could tell him about Mark that no one else would know. Joey shared what he knew.

Several weeks later, Robert had the opportunity to fly to the east coast where Mark lived. Wanting to test the authenticity of the Joey encounter, Robert asked Mark if he was training the dog to get him a beer out of the cooler, which was one of the statements Joey had made. Mark was surprised Robert knew that. They were both amazed by the other things Joey had conveyed to Robert that were equally accurate.

Robert proceeded to place Mark in a hypnotic trance. Like Antoinette, he too was able to perceive and communicate with Joey. They asked Joey if he could tell them five things concerning Antoinette that no one else would know. Robert returned to San Diego, CA and relayed the information to Antoinette. She was quite shocked at the personal nature of what Joey knew about her and impressed that he was able to clearly share it with Mark. This experience helped Robert recognize new and exciting possibilities for his hypnosis work.

Robert set up a meeting for the following week with Antoinette at her home. He wanted to explore her ability to communicate with other spirits while in a hypnotic trance. During that meeting, Antoinette's friend Sam was in the room. He was not in hypnotic trance but appeared to communicate with spirits as well. This was completely unexpected and awed everyone present. Robert was fascinated by this and asked Sam and Antoinette to come to his house to test Sam's skill under trance.

Robert had just read the book entitled *Into The Wild* by Jon Krakauer. Synopsis:

> In April 1992 a young man from a well-to-do family hitchhiked to Alaska and walked alone into the wilderness north of Mt. McKinley. His name was Christopher Johnson McCandless. He had given $25,000 in savings to charity, abandoned his car and most of his possessions, burned all the cash in his wallet, and invented a new life for himself. Four months later, his decomposed body was found by a moose hunter. How McCandless came to die is the unforgettable story of *Into the Wild.*[2]

---

[2] Source for Into The Wild by Jon Krakauer book summary is Amazon.com.

Robert knew Sam had not read the book. He decided to test Sam's ability by calling in the spirit of Chris McCandless who did come through. Sam was able to communicate with him for about forty five minutes. Chris explained his passing was in response to a karmic debt. Before closing the session, Robert asked Chris what he could do for him. Sam relayed the reply: "Contact my sister because she cries for me every day." Then he gave several personal messages to relay to Chris's sister, Carine.

"That's great Chris," Robert communicated through Sam. "But you've been dead a long time. How would your sister know the communication is from you?" Without hesitation, through Sam, Chris relayed a secret that only Carine and Chris knew. Robert was able to phone Carine the following Monday and relay Chris's secret message. She replied, "Only Chris and I know about that!" Out of respect for Carine's privacy we will not state the details of that message. However, Carine concurred that the message was indeed from Chris.

Over the next year Chris' messages were relayed through Sam to Carine. In time Carine decided to fly out to San Diego with a friend. I was able to observe as she communicated directly with Chris through Sam. After a long talk, Carine asked Chris if he was aware that there were people who wanted to make a movie about his life based on the book written about him by Jon Krakauer. Chris did know about it. Carine asked Chris if he was okay with that. Chris replied that he wanted the movie to be made with some suggestions for it that he provided that day.

To my knowledge movie director Sean Penn was not

apprised of the mediumship involved in the family finally making the decision to authorize his making of the movie. It was Chris's feeling that releasing this information prior to or at the time of the movie's release might take away from the other messages that he wanted portrayed in the movie. However, Jon Krakauer was told about it and phoned Robert to discuss it.

From that point forward, Antoinette and Sam got together twice a week with Robert. There were all types of communications with a host of spirits of the deceased who could offer insight regarding one topic or another. People would gather to communicate with deceased family and friends through Sam. In some instances they pursued missing person cases via help from deceased ancestors or the diseased themselves. Other guests at the sessions would learn about past lives, spirit guides and even health issues through Antoinette. During that time, Robert also held private sessions for people that wanted to explore their metaphysical abilities under hypnotic trance. During those early years there were no holds barred.

I learned several key things from observing. First, the talents or interests a person pursues in this life often are areas they can tap into while in trance for additional insights. The instance that stands out the most is when a man in his late thirties named Dave wanted to explore his capabilities. None of us were aware of his keen interest in the weather. But we discovered that he could describe upcoming weather patterns. That year there was an extreme heat wave in Texas. Dave went into trance one day and predicted the exact high temperature for each day of the upcoming forty days or so for a town afflicted by the high temperatures. He even identified the day the heat wave would break. No one knew what to do with the information and so we moved on to other things.

One important key element to all of what was transpiring can be summed up in the word 'modulation'. It is the term used to describe attuning or calibrating one's personal vibration to the frequency of a particular spirit realm. The concept of modulation is easier for most people to understand in relation to musical notes or mantras because we actually calibrate to sound all the time. But it is also true of accessing spirit realms. Like a singer who exercises their voice by practicing singing the notes on a musical scale, one too, can practice 'modulating' to attune to a different wavelength.

So in 2012 when I got *Attached*, the **only** people I knew aware of and working to clear *Attachments* were Robert and his Ghost Remover team. They are the only spiritual workers that I'm familiar with that can modulate successfully into and out of the spaces between the realms where ghosts are stuck. Of course, as I was to discover, there is much more to it than modulation.

Testing the boundaries of what was possible, there was a time when famous people were summoned because Sam was so good at modulating into or accessing the realms they resided in. Humble and private in regards to his talent, I find he is the best medium (also known as necromancer) that I have ever encountered.

During one session, Sam relayed the information that leaders transition to a special place for further development because they influence so many people. Though many were contacted, I recall in particular the communication with ex-president Jefferson because I was impressed by his insights. He said that one thing that always amazed him was that no matter how good intentioned he or a proposal was for the people that about half the people would be for it and half against it. Eventually, he came to anticipate this division.

In another case, a forty-five year old professional sound recorder named Bill wanted to explore his past lives and meet his guide while under trance. He was able to do that and discovered a vital connection between one past life in particular that influenced him in this life. That is a common occurrence. But what was most memorable to me was when Robert asked Bill's guide who on the other side might be helpful to his work. The guide replied, Joseph Campbell, who of course Robert was already familiar with. She then mentioned a second name unfamiliar to us all; H.P. The Voice of the Silence. I didn't make much note of it at the time. Bill went home and looked up the information about his guide and his past life. He was able to find reference to the historical places and events he learned about during the session. Those were fascinating to him. But what caught my attention was when he returned to report that he had looked up H.P. and learned that was a reference to a person called Helena Blavatsky.

Helena Petrovna Blavatsky was an occultist, spirit medium, and author who co-founded the Theosophical Society in 1875. She gained an international following as the leading theoretician of Theosophy, the esoteric movement that the Society promoted. The Theosophical Society had once had a center in Point Loma, CA.

There were many such cases in which information came through a session that one or more of us would be interested in. These were vital leads for the seekers who came to the sessions. In other cases, there came advice to intervene. In this next case, Robert and Antoinette learn that spirit guides are an underutilized resource in the pursuit of freeing troubled people from past life influence.

SESSION: A New Spirit Guide

Robert writes about how they met:

> Antoinette was a caretaker at the time for Mark, a paraplegic. She had brought Mark to our session that day so that we could inquire with the spirit realm to find out if there was anything we might do to help him.

> However, while my sister Antoinette was in a trance state a new voice spoke through her. The voice introduced herself. "Hello, my name is Rajah and I want to speak to you about Mark, is that all right with you?" "Yes." I replied. Rajah then continued, "Before we proceed I have to get permission." We waited for a few moments for Rajah to return. I'd imagine that she went up some spiritual chain of command. Apparently she went up to a God level because when Rajah returned she told us; "Alright, I have permission to speak through your sister."

> Of course my first question was "Who gives you permission?" In a matter-of-fact manner Rajah answers "God of course. He is the only one who can." This was the first time a spirit obtained permission to communicate but it was not the last.

Rajah and I go on to discuss Mark's situation. We learn from Rajah that she knew him during a past life many hundreds of years ago. She explained that they had lived back then as husband and wife. In that life, Mark was found guilty of stealing. His punishment was being blinded in one eye, his right arm and both his legs broken. *Because he did not forgive himself*, he recreated the same injuries in the skateboarding accident he incurred as a teenager in this life which has left him wheelchair bound.

She goes on to explain, "It has been a long time since I walked the earth. We lived in much simpler time then. I lived a special life. I had a great family and fond memories of that experience. I only had the one life and when I returned back home to the spirit world I decided to stay. In time, I became head of the spirit guides. I love my position."

She continues; "Everyone on earth is a spirit having a physical experience." "Everyone has a spirit guide then?" I asked. "Yes. Some people have more than one. It all depends on what that person is doing on earth. If the guides are interested in what they are doing they might have four or five guides. It all depends upon the nature of their pursuits. Then there other occasions where one guide watches over more than one person at a time."

"You Robert, have one guide. He goes by the name of Caleb. He was your best friend from Greece in your last life. You and he stowed away on a ship to America. The ship was caught in a storm and sank. You drowned but your friend did not. He was able to save himself by holding on to a part of the wreckage to stay above water. You, however, have drowned in many of your past lives. I don't know why you still go in the water so much." (I live near and often swim in the Pacific ocean.) "I certainly wouldn't." quips Rajah. "In fact, once you drowned in two feet of water. You were a fisherman in Mexico who had too much to drink. As a result you fell and hit your head on a rock and drowned. There are other stories but we will save them for another time. You have lived many lives. Thirty two to be exact. That is a lot."

Rajah changes the subject. "I check in on Mark and I'm concerned about the way in which he is being mistreated at the hands of others while he is at his home." I ask what we can do for Mark. "There is nothing we can do for Mark at the moment." Rajah said. "I will give you the guidance to perform a healing on Mark in the near future. The essence of the ceremony will be on forgiveness. He needs to forgive himself for his actions in that past life so that he does not carry it forward yet again into another future life."

Rajah adds, "I will come back if you want me to and teach you many things. All you have to do is put Antoinette in trance and I will come." I replied, "That would be fantastic Rajah. I'm sure Antoinette will want to do this. Can she hear the conversation you and I are having now?" I asked. "Partially." Rajah replied. "She is outside of her body but is aware of what is happening while I'm in her body. She cannot stay out of her body too long.

It is time for me to say goodbye and for her to return to her body."

Rajah became their main teacher regarding information about the spirit world in general. Their communications were invaluable. Additionally, they provided the necessary information that laid the foundation for and answered many questions during future explorations. They first learned about *Attachments* from her while working with a married man and father of two children named Saul.

Since his twenties Saul had struggled with alcoholism. Now in his forties, no matter how much he tried to change the course in his life, bad things happened to Saul on a continuous basis. He was having more than an average person's share of accidents and altercations. As a result, Robert decided to consult Rajah about his situation.

Rajah informed Robert that Saul was not struggling from past life issues as in the case of Mark. Instead, Saul was in fact, *Attached*. This was the first time Robert had heard that reference from Rajah. Robert was astonished by this revelation and endeavored to learn all he could about the problem. He wanted to know how *Attachments* adversely affected his clients and what could be done about it. He discovered that earthbound spirits, also known as ghosts, can *Attach* themselves to anyone. While connected to that person they can greatly disrupt the natural flow of a person's life. And, it was an *Attachment* that was the source of Saul's problems.

A ghost is the spirit of someone (person or animal) who has lived a life on earth and remains earthbound. For whatever reason, they become confused or disoriented at or just after the time of death. This results in their becoming lost in transition. These beings are anyone's ancestors, siblings, even offspring. They are not necessarily evil as some would have you believe. There are a good percentage of them that don't bother anybody else at all. But there are others that do. And when they do, that is when Rajah refers to them as *Attachments*.

During the next few weeks Robert assembled a team of people as directed by Rajah that would be required to remove the *Attachment*. In preparation for the removal she gave instructions in advance to Robert. This initial removal session included gathering items as well. Among them were flower essences and crystals.

Robert assembled his team. A group of people gathered to watch the new process. There was a lot of anticipation and excitement emanating from the people present. Saul arrived. Rajah's instructions were followed to the letter. Rajah instructed and guided the team throughout the process. In retrospect, much of the guidance was most similar to the practice of exorcism.

This initial *Attachment* removal was a lengthy ordeal. It took about an hour. When the *Attachment* finally released its grip on Saul and was detached, it departed. As it did, all the windows in the place shook. The observers who gathered to watch that were seated on the sofa and chairs nearest the door got up and fled the place in fright. They gathered outside until they calmed themselves down enough to come back inside.

Since that first removal, Rajah, other spirit guides, Robert and the Ghost Remover team have perfected and streamlined the process into what it is today. However, they continue to rely on Rajah's gracious guidance. At times, she comes in on her own accord with information that helps them with their work.

There have been many, many cases since that first removal which is now over eighteen years ago. Robert and his team have experienced amazing revelations and are always receiving new information from the spirit world. Each case the Ghost Remover team works on expands their knowledge and extends their abilities to help others. Their removal process has grown and evolved to cope with the many different scenarios that they encounter today. The material in this book combined with Robert Major's actual case files endeavors to provide an overview of the nature of this problem.

Case File clients are referred to by first names only (and often those are pseudonyms) to maintain their privacy. Aspects of what they have experienced are presented in this book. It is my hope that for those readers who recognize that their experiences are similar to the ones expressed within these pages, like me, they can finally identify the source of their affliction and recognize the possibility of a solution.

In an effort to share what Robert and his team now know I find that the complex nature of being human is much more dimensional than it appears to be. Living people are interacting with the spirit world all of the time and in different ways. They have spirit helpers who are constantly trying to guide them, and they can become enmeshed with wandering earthbound spirits that are no longer alive, but have not moved on to the other realms. Robert is dedicated to helping people that have problems arising from these types of entanglements. His view of the world and our place within it is forever changing and so are the lives of the people he encounters.

CHAPTER 2:
SPIRIT COMMUNICATION AND BEYOND

This chapter presents a sampling of the myriad of Ghost Remover spirit communications that have taken place sometime during the last two decades. Each encounter is unique. Nevertheless, these sessions offer distinctive insights into the complex nature of the relationship between the living and the spirit realm.

In this next account of a session, Robert became aware of details about circumstances relating to an unsolved missing person's case.

SESSION entitled: The Case of a Missing College Student.

The Ghost Remover team was in communication with the spirit of a missing deceased college-aged student. Given the situation he was in just prior to his death, he tells them he was incapacitated and then murdered. Therefore, he could not give much information beyond the names of the three perpetrators. That is not evidence enough to offer any kind of lead usable to the police to act upon. Spirit guide communications indicated that there was a deceased relative present at the time of the incident.

Robert Major wrote a letter to the authorities working on the case to share the information the victim provided in the hopes it could help the authorities working on the case. The police responded because there was information in his letter that was purposely withheld by police. After several conversations, Robert asked them for and received the information needed to summon the victim's deceased grandfather. Without the man's name and date of birth there is the possibility for an imposter to respond to the summons. It is better to be as specific as possible.

During the session with the grandfather, much was learned about what happened that night. He was far more descriptive of the events and where they took place because of his unique vantage point at the time. He says that he was hovering just above what was happening whereas his grandson was incapacitated and had his eyes covered.

Robert took note of the information provided and followed the leads about 160 miles north of San Diego to the location where it was indicated that the body had been buried years before. While he and his team could clearly find the markers identified by the grandfather they could not find the body in the heavily wooded area. Without the body, the police case to this day remains as a missing person.

The Ghost Removers returned to Robert's home and opened up a channel to the spirit realm to inquire about what they had missed during their search. However, a spirit entity stepped in and advised the team that there were other things that needed to play out in this situation. He told them that they were not to proceed further because it could interfere with upcoming events that needed to play out first. The spirit assured them that all will come out to resolve this mystery after a few other things happened to the perpetrators. The Ghost Removers adhered to this guidance. Rarely do divine spirits intervene in such a manner, but it does happen.

From the case just described and others like it, it becomes apparent that deceased family and friends watch over us while we're alive. The familial ties are not cut at death. Therefore, it only makes sense that family members that predecease us are there to greet us when we pass-over into the other side as well as to young children who are acclimating to their earthly surroundings.

The next presentation is of a different nature. It is the story of Ruth Ellis, a spirit guide. It is from the early years during which there were many such cases in which information came through a session that one or more of those present would be interested in. These were vital leads for the seekers who came to the sessions. In other cases, there came advice to intervene.

It is generally accepted in western spiritualism that a spirit guide is an entity that remains as a disincarnate spirit to act as a guide or protector to a living incarnated human being. Some spirit guides are persons who have lived many former lifetimes, paid their karmic debts, and advanced beyond a need to reincarnate.

Many devotees believe that spirit guides are chosen on "the other side" by human beings who are about to incarnate and wish assistance. Spirit guides often desire guiding or teaching the living in areas of common interest or pursuits. Sometimes a spirit guide can inspire a person to notice or take interest in something new. In other cases, one or more new spirit guides come to someone who is ready to take their passion to a new level.

Spirit guides employ the same mechanisms that ghosts use to communicate to the living. The difference is intention. Spirit guides destine, meaning they choose someone for a particular purpose or end, for the benefit of that person. Or, as in the case of a leader, they seek to influence for the greater good overall.

Ruth Ellis made herself known to Robert Major rather unexpectedly during an ordinary session with their spirit guide Rajah. Robert found that the more he communicated into these realms, the more those who wanted to communicate from the spirit world found him. In time, instead of summoning them, they began to appear of their own accord.

The following is a case file from Robert's archives that demonstrates how a spirit guide can help the living.

SESSION: <u>More than a Vehicle Transaction</u>

Robert Major recalls:

> A number of years ago while in session we were speaking in our customary manner with a spirit guide Rajah when we were interrupted. She asked us if it was all right if the woman who was breaking into our communication could speak. Apparently she believed that her message was urgent. Our guide said that she was holding a red flag to express that what she had to say was extremely urgent.

From our experience this was totally out of the ordinary and so we agreed to let her speak feeling it must be important. This female spirit quickly entered the communication and introduced herself through Antoinette saying, "Hello. My name is Ruth Ellis."

In a hurried manner Ms. Ellis explained, "I was the last woman hanged in Holloway prison. I murdered my boyfriend in a jealous rage and I was hanged for it. It is very important that I speak with you. I am the guide of the woman you met yesterday. She came to your house with her husband and sat right there. Antoinette's arm raises and points to the place on the sofa where the woman had indeed sat the day before. But even without that I knew who she meant.

I had sold a big old white Ford truck meant for hauling to a gentleman the day before. He brought his wife along to drive his vehicle back home while he drove the truck. I remembered her name was Pam. Ruth said, "You must stop her. She is thinking of committing suicide and I cannot let that happen. As her guide, I am responsible for her. You must speak to her and tell her not to do it. It will cost her dearly." "I can call her." I said. "But she may think I'm a little out there with regards to how I got this information."

Before proceeding further I asked Ruth how she ended up as a guide if she had murdered someone. "Didn't you have to pay for such an act?" I asked. She said, "I paid dearly. Not only was I hanged for the murder but I had to return two more times and die two horrible deaths as a child. Plus my own son killed himself when he was a young man so you see it all ties together. My actions affected so many people. That's why I feel so distressed right now. I need your help." I told her that I would call Pam right away once we were finished with our session and talk to her about this.

I have made a number of these phone calls and written letters on behalf of spirits many times. Even if it falls on deaf ears I still do it. In Pam's case I had to call her husband's number and ask to speak to his wife. That was somewhat awkward but I did it. I reintroduced myself to Pam as the man who sold her husband the truck. I went on to tell her that I was a hypnotist who dealt with the paranormal. And, during a session we had just concluded I received some information that she was considering suicide. I told her the spirit world refers to suicide as "a permanent solution to a temporary problem". They go on to say that all things will pass and to just give it time.

There was a pause during which neither of us spoke. It was followed by a flood of expression as Pam poured out her woes to me. Pam relayed to me just how life had overwhelmed her lately. And, that even though she was thinking of suicide she didn't believe she would actually follow through with it.

I shared with Pam a few of the stories I knew of about those who have committed suicide. When I checked on them through spirit connections I was told that they ended up in a solitary darkness for a very long time. That is if they even cross over into the light. If they don't they become part of the walking dead here on earth. That creates even bigger problems for themselves.

As our conversation drew to a close, Pam assured me she would work through things instead of contemplating suicide. She thanked me for my concern. I hung up the phone hoping that the call made a difference.

Afterwards I went online and looked up Ruth Ellis. There she was, "The last woman hanged in England in 1955." It turns out that Ruth was quite famous for that and that a movie was made about her story. She did have to pay for her misdeeds but she is alright now.

It is not the first time that spirit communication has revealed that being sorry or apologizing does not always result in forgiveness. In Ruth's case, it was an eye for an eye and a tooth for a tooth. It was just in her next lives that she paid the price for her behavior. And having learned from these experiences, Ruth is now a spirit guide that helps others facing life and death choices. Ruth can guide living human beings in these regards because she has first-hand experience in this situation.

A google search on the name Ruth Ellis brings up a lot of resources. According to the article entitled *The Tragic Story of Ruth Ellis, The Las Woman Hanged in Britain* by

Kara Goldfarb, Published March 12, 2018 In 1955, Ruth Ellis was hanged for shooting her lover. Her execution sparked a public conversation that would ultimately lead to the abolishment of the death penalty. The article portrayed this photograph.

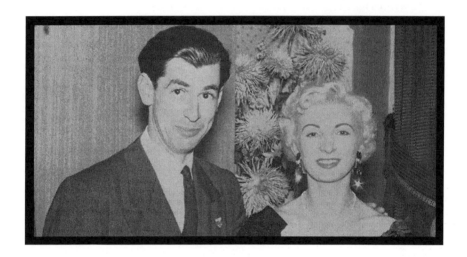

Getty Images of Racecar driver David Blakely with Ruth Ellis, a 28-year-old model and mother of two. Ellis, who was having an affair with Blakely, shot and killed him as he exited a pub with his friends.

One might wonder how a convicted murderess could become a spirit guide to the living. The answer lies in a philosophy most of us have heard at one time or another. That is, Earth is a school. Every school comes with its set of tests and lessons. Therefore, every experience we have in life is a Spiritual test and lesson to demonstrate our Divinity in thought, in feeling, in word, and in physical action and deed.

Experiences are opportunities to learn and grow. The spiritual philosophy pertaining to the earth school is that if we learn our lessons, we don't have to reincarnate any more. However, if we fail a lesson, we have to repeat the class in this life or the next.

It has been said that experience is the best teacher. There is a Chinese Proverb that says "Only He who has travelled the road knows where the holes are deep."

Whether in this life or the next, people are given an opportunity to learn and grow from their misdeeds. Ruth has evolved to a point now where she is a Spirit Guide who does what she can to help living people who are experiencing troubled times make healthier choices.

At or around the time of death, many people successfully transition to the afterlife. However, some do not. There are many reasons why a person fails to make the transition. Interestingly, Robert Major has come across many instances where the deceased chose to ghost because of their belief in the grave as being *their final resting place.*

Robert Major finds that the beliefs in where someone goes in the afterlife varies greatly. "I am not here to debate where a person goes after they die." He says. "My concern is for those that are stuck here. These are the spirits that we encounter every day. They need help to move on. Sometimes they end up being your deceased family or friends that get lost in transition. Other times, they are relatives or friends of someone else. They are not devils. They are not evil spirits. They are often disoriented and disconnected from this life and their new place in the afterlife. They inhabit a void in between worlds in an unnatural state of being. In other cases, they have unfinished business with the living. In these cases, they chose the 'void' in between worlds instead of moving on deliberately as a means of continuing a pursuit or cause."

That being said, in contrast to the Abrahamic tradition of the afterlife being determined by a deity, in systems of reincarnation, such as those in the Dharmic tradition, the nature of continued existence is determined directly by the actions of the individual in the ended life, rather than through the decision of another being. Under these conditions the individual may be reborn into this world and begin the life cycle over again, likely with no memory of what they have done in the past. In this view, such rebirths and deaths may take place over and over again continuously until the individual gains entry to a spiritual realm or otherworld. The next incident is a fascinating account on the topic of karma.

SESSION: *He* was to be a Woman who Knows Nothing
Robert Major recalls:

> "Her real name, interestingly, is JoAnne. Joe is typically a man's name. Anne, a feminine designation. JoAnne was a young girl of about fifteen years of age at the time. I knew some of her personal history. Her biological parents had been big drinkers. As a result, JoAnne was born with fetal alcohol syndrome. Her mother died shortly after giving birth. Her father had since passed. JoAnne lived with a couple who were paid to be her caretakers."

> "JoAnne was short, about five feet tall and chubby.

Even though she was born female, she already had traces of a beard. By all outward appearances, one could not identify if she was male or female. She spoke quite unintelligibly and anytime she got around anybody, she always seemed desperate for attention."

"While in session one day speaking with Rajah, JoAnne who lived down the street from Antoinette at the time, came knocking at the door. I answered and told her she would have to come back later because we were in session. As I spoke to her I thought how sad to be born like that and how hard her life must be."

"It occurred to me to ask Rajah, 'Is there something we can do for that girl? She has so many problems'." Rajah replied much faster than I anticipated. "No. You are not to intervene. She was born that way for a reason. You see, in a previous life she was a man. He lived in the land known as Serbia and was part of the military there. He would use his position of authority to rape young women. He was ruthless. So in this life, he was to be born a woman who knows nothing. That is his karmic debt he is paying for and there is nothing you can do to help. Her parents that gave birth to her have passed on. They did not have to karmicly care for her for her entire life. The caretakers are well paid and happy for the opportunity to do the job. In these ways, JoAnne is isolated at nobody else's expense. And, she is to be a man who lives in a woman's body. There is nothing you can do to help her." That was a lesson for me that day and I began to see the world in a clearer light.

There have been other instances where it was revealed that karma played a role in a person's current life. Beyond that, Robert has hypnotized people who expressed an interest in exploring one or more past lives to uncover influences in that that lifetime that affect them now.

Past Life Regression is a technique that uses hypnosis to recover memories or experiences of past lives or incarnations. Past life explanations help validate what physicists theorize today, that is we humans are not totally bound by time and space.

Hypnotherapist Robert Major's case files are rich with past life client file accounts that have threads woven their way into current life issues. Upon making the connection between past and current lives, evokes a kind of *healing* through understanding for clients. Here's one example.

SESSION: An uncontrollable urge to smoke. . .
In the case of this 40 year old female client, she came to Robert Major because she wanted to stop smoking cigarettes. She'd been smoking since a teenager and had tried to quit many times since but was unsuccessful. Robert used a hypnotic induction to place the client into a hypnotic trance state. From there, Robert asked the client to recall the first time she ever wanted a cigarette. To his amazement, the client responded quite emphatically that she was five years old. His experience led him to regress this client into a past life where she smoked. Whether the

link to smoking in the past life was so strong or the client was simply adept, she shifted into the past life and into the personality of the cowboy she was back then. Her facial expression, posturing and tone of voice all changed as well. The client leaned forward a bit, squinted while looking at her hands making the motion of rolling an invisible cigarette. "I used to roll them with one hand." the client stated in a type of deep voice rich in country western drawl. With the connection made between the role of cigarette smoking in past and present lives, the client was able to eventually kick the habit. Though it was a challenge, she did it. As of this writing she has not smoked in over a decade.

In time, Robert and his team have found their spirit guides provide easy access to past lives including significant lifetime and affects from past lives that have an effect on a person in this lifetime. For instance, though rare amongst Ghost Remover case files, there are instances where a ghost who was able to attach itself to the client made the transition from a client's past life to their current one. They cleared the client of the ghost (referred to as an *Attachment*) and the presenting issues it brought with it likewise cleared from her life.

In this next case, a middle-aged man's past life influence was of a different nature. For the most part, the type of ghosting state a spirit may end up in and the location that it haunts is in direct relation to where the person was when he died. However, that standard does not apply when there is a case of unfinished business. There have been many cases in which ghosts from the past have tracked down others from their time that are reincarnated and living now.

In this particular case, spirits tracked down a man to apologize for a past life incident.

CASE FILE: The Apology

Several years ago, while Robert was interested in and involved with people who were conducting residential energy efficiency audits in the state of California, he met a man named Jason. Jason was in his early thirties. He was a qualified inspector who performed energy efficiency audits.

Robert had known Jason about three months when, during a session, a Spirit by the name of Chief Porcupine Bear asked to be re-united with Jason who he stated was his cousin during a previous life when they were dog soldiers. Chief Porcupine Bear wanted to speak to his cousin. When he made this request, he said he'd been seeking a means to communicate with Jason and asked Robert if he would summon Jason to a session the following week. Robert agreed.

Robert revealed to Jason that he and his team had spiritual connections and communicated regularly with the spirit realm. Robert explained to Jason that his presence was requested at the next session. Jason agreed to attend.

As the session opened, Antoinette explained that the communication posed challenges because of translating between languages. The following is a condensed version of the transcript.

Many Native Americans in spirit gathered for the

session but only Chief Porcupine Bear came through in the session to speak. "We've been tracking Little Creek but not found him up until now. This is a great disguise (pointing to Jason's body and inferring he's a white man.)" He continues his communication by saying that he wants to say he is sorry for mortally wounding his cousin Little Creek, who is now Jason. He goes on to explain that even though his other cousin, Around, was involved that it was actually his stabbing that killed him. Little Creek, now Jason, was stabbed many times in the chest by both men. However, it was he, Chief Porcupine Bear that gave him the mortal wound to the heart. It appeared to others that he had Around finish him off and that is what is alleged[3] but that's not what killed Little

---

[3] Post session research identified this account of the encounter: Prior to the peace council held at Bent's Fort in 1840, the Algonquian-speaking Southern Cheyenne and Arapaho were allied against their traditional enemies, the Comanche, Kiowa, and Plains Apache, who belonged to different language families and cultures. In 1837, while raiding the Kiowa horse herds along the North Fork of the Red River, a party of 48 Cheyenne Bowstring Men were discovered and killed by Kiowa and Comanche warriors. Porcupine Bear, chief of the Dog Soldiers, took up the war pipe of the Cheyenne. He carried it to the various Cheyenne and Arapaho camps to drum up support for revenge against the Kiowa. He reached a Northern Cheyenne camp along the South Platte River just after it had traded liquor from American Fur Company men at Fort Laramie.
Porcupine Bear joined in the drinking. He sat and sang Dog Soldier war songs. Two of his cousins, Little Creek and Around, became caught up in a drunken fight. Little Creek got on top of Around and held up a knife, ready to stab Around; at that point, Porcupine Bear, aroused by Around's calls for help, tore the knife away from Little Creek, and stabbed him with it several times. He forced Around to finish off Little Creek.

Creek. He killed him. So he is apologizing.

Little Creek was Chief Porcupine Bear's mother's sister's child. Another cousin, Around, was with Chief Porcupine Bear in spirit during the session but did not speak. Robert asked questions and Chief Porcupine Bear answered them. Here is a summary of what he had to say:

The important thing to him is this apology. He is apologizing for the death of Little Creek. Chief Porcupine Bear explained why he killed Little Creek. He states that he had been drinking very heavily. "You (Little Creek) were fighting with Around (your cousin) and I told you boys to stop. It was a family fight."

They were dog soldiers at the time, referred to by the whites as Hotamintaneo (Hotamin for short). Both Chief Porcupine Bear and Little Creek were very tough. They protected their own people as well as others. Little Creek survived many 'pinnings'.[4] Chief Porcupine Bear explains that the

---

By the rules governing military societies, a man who murdered or accidentally killed another tribe member had blood on his hands and was prohibited from joining a society. A society member who committed such a crime was expelled and outlawed. Porcupine Bear was expelled from the Dog Soldiers, and he and his relatives had to camp apart from the rest of the Cheyenne. The Dog Soldiers were disgraced by Porcupine Bear's act. The other chiefs forbade them from leading war against the Kiowa. Source: https://en.wikipedia.org/wiki/Dog_Soldiers October 3, 2016

[4] Post session research resulted in this finding the following reference:
Attached to each dog rope was a picket-pin used to tether horses. The pin was driven into the ground as a mark of resolve in combat. When a dog soldier was

custom is to pin oneself to the ground and stay there until another soldier relieves them or until they get slain. Little Creek is significant because he survived many 'pinnings'. It's not a good life. But that's the tradition. They fought everybody, Indians and White People alike. It had been just after a raid.

After that incident they were ousted from the Cheyenne tribe for killing one of their own. They had to camp outside the tribe. "I didn't drink after that day. I never drank again.", he said.

Robert comments, there are not many opportunities nowadays for Native warriors to fight. "Not true." Replies Chief Porcupine Bear. "They fight in your wars."

Chief Porcupine Bear wanted to know "Why did you (Jason) come back like that?" (meaning white) What was it that led to the choice to do so? Robert interjected that Jason would not have access to that knowledge, they would have to learn that later. Chief Porcupine Bear asked Little Creek (Jason) to join them in the spirit world. He asks if Little Creek

---

staked to the ground in order to cover the retreat of his companions, he was required to remain there even if death was the consequence. The Dog Man could pull the pin from the ground only if his companions reached safety or another Dog Soldier released him from his duties. Source: www.manataka.org page 164.

would consider body-hopping out and letting another spirit have the body. Robert interjects that Jason has a wife and children and that this is his life now. The spirits that came to the session turned to depart and said 'goodbye' as they left.

Robert then asked Jason for his comments about the session. Here is what Jason had to say:

"I've had different dreams where I can see a man as a Chief. He's an older gentleman, and there's a group, a congregation with him as he's chanting and I'm on the outside of the group. I'm paying attention to him but he's not really paying attention to me. He's paying attention to the people he's sitting with. And as soon as he pays attention to me, I wake up."

"And, I've also had dreams where I'm in a hot spring or a hot tub and I'm relaxing and it's definitely a middle aged Indian that comes down while I'm relaxing and stabs me in the chest repeatedly. And, I'm still alive. Like he can't kill me. He's stabbing and stabbing and stabbing and I'm serene in this pool. I was already serene in the pool and there's no movement by me to try to even stop him. I just kind of go. And wake."

In this case, the communication was made first and foremost to make the apology for the stabbing of Little Creek that resulted in his death. Robert considers this an example of a case of additional unfinished business because the spirits clearly communicated their desire that Little Creek (now Jason) leave his body behind and join them in the spirit world.

The Ghost Removers are a new and revolutionary type of team because they deal with ghosts. They recognize both the helping nature as well as the unwanted influence of a spirit as destructive to a person's well being.

Based on certain beliefs, some may think that the voices of the dead are all around us, when in fact, they are the spirits of the dead themselves. These spirits may have become lost or confused just after death, or they have chosen not to move on because they feel they have unfinished business and are still trying to interact with us. Some of them co-exist with the living. Some of these interactions are benevolent, even playful, while others can be disturbing or harmful. It is this complex nature of the spirit realm that makes it fascinating.

But because of the mainstream climate here in the West, if by chance you perceive or hear them and report what you see, your experience will often be discredited as hallucinations that are *'all in your mind.'* Robert Major and his team do not discount these experiences or the person report them. They know from experience that it is in fact spirit entities. Ghost Removers can confirm the presence of helping spirit guides as well as the problems associated with involuntary spirit influence from ghosts. These experiences are very real.

CHAPTER 3:
BECOMING EARTHBOUND

A person's spirit is the part of their being that can transcend the physical self. It moves on from this life into the afterlife. However, it is not always a smooth transition to the higher realms. Spirit's of people that have just died can become confused or not understand that they have indeed died. Perhaps they died suddenly, as in an accident. Or perhaps they do not want to move on for some compelling reason. These spirits are lost and have failed to make it to their true destination in the afterlife. The following session is one example of how this could happen.

SESSION: When in Trouble, Stay Put!
Robert Major recalls:

"Sometimes we get an instinct about a situation and follow-up on it." Says Robert. "For instance, there was a car accident on a Southern California freeway where the teenage girl driver died. Her vehicle was rear ended while driving on the freeway. Based upon my hunch that something was amiss, I checked on her through our spirit connections. We found that the teenager was ghosting at the scene of the accident because she was waiting for her mom to come and get her.

As is often the case, I contact a family member to let them know what we do and offer the means to communicate to the deceased. In this case, I mailed a letter to the teenagers mother. A few days my roommate arrives home and found a checkbook on the front doorstop. I called the owner of the checks and learned that she was the mother of the driver. Too distraught to phone me back, she decided to visit me instead. When I wasn't at home she began to have second thoughts about showing up unannounced and must have dropped her checkbook on the front stoop when retrieving her car keys from her purse. In time, we were able to get the two in contact with each other and set the daughter free.

Her mother communicated to me that she had always told her that if she ever got into trouble to stay put until she arrived. In this case, she did. Additionally, her mother said that she gained closure as a result of communicating with her daughter and guiding her to go safely on her way into the next world. And, she was especially impressed by the intimate messages transmitted through Sam the Necromancer. Without his ability to transmit details no one else would know from her daughter to her, she would not have responded to the opportunity to communicate through him with her daughter in the first place."

Afterlife is the general term used when referring to the time that begins at the moment of death. It is the concept of a realm, or the realm itself (whether physical or transcendental), in which an essential part of an individual's identity or consciousness continues to exist after the death of the physical body. Death can occur as a result of accident or in other ways.

Throughout history people have turned to drugs for medicinal or recreational purposes. In more recent times there are various drugs used for many different reasons. The current trending substances of concern are Opioids. It is reported by the 2016 US National Survey on Drug Use and Health that 116 people die every day from Opioid related drug overdoses.

Up next: **CASE FILE:** #0111 *The Case of The Accidental Overdose.* It is about an experiment with drugs that lead to an unfortunate turn of events. The following is a transcript of the case.

Robert: This next case involves a referral to inquire if a newly deceased young man is ghosting. We checked on him through our spirit guide and learned that he is indeed ghosting. Therefore, we are here today parked outside of his home to investigate further and find out if we can help the young man find peace.

What we know at this point is that the young man is believed to have fallen victim to the Opioid crisis.

Beyond that, what I can tell you is the people involved want to remain anonymous. Therefore, we will not disclose any specific details which might reveal their identities. To do that, we are filming on location from inside our vehicle. Join us now as we explore this case further.

Robert: What's going to happen is that Antoinette is going to go into trance. Then, she will bring in her spirit guide Lane. He will detail for us what is actually happening here.

Antoinette: My initial impression is that the ghost of the young man is only about 500 feet away from where we are parked by his house. Now, I will go into trance.

Robert: Antoinette is now in trance. Now, spirit guide Lane is present. He's going to help us with what we do today.

Spirit Guide Lane: We are going to do a type of 'ghost intervention'. But for now, I'm going to step aside and let Antoinette back in so she can communicate what goes on.

Antoinette: He (the newly deceased) is inside the house. He knows that we are here to move him. He is coming out of his house to the car. *After a pause* . . . He's here (just outside the car window to Antoinette's right). He is conveying to me that he is distraught. He's showing me that he is very sad for his family. He wants us to know that he *did not* commit suicide.

41

Robert: We did not think you did.

Antoinette: He's saying that he was just experimenting (with drugs) because he was so busy in his head all the time that he was not getting any sleep.

Robert: What drugs did you experiment with? Were they tainted?

Antoinette shifts to allowing the young man speak for himself in answer to Robert's question.

Young Man: No. I took three different kinds and my body disagreed.

Robert: We're sad for you.

Young Man: Well Yeah. I was too young! Man, I had a life. I had an opportunity to go into this smoky green colored opening that I saw. There was a female family member calling to me. I didn't go because I didn't know what it was. And, I wasn't really sure that I was (deceased) because I was in-between. Now, I'm fully understanding that I was in-between meaning either staying here with my mom or going. She feels like she's going to die (from grief). Now, I don't know where to go.

Note: The session is disrupted by this author's phone ringing. These types of disruptions cause spirits duress because it is of a loud pitch that does has an adverse effect on the plane they exist on. In this case, the sound initially scared the young man. Spirits often cut off the communication temporarily and did so in this case. Afterwards the young man described the sound as 'pitchy' to him.

Antoinette: The young man has left and we'll try to get him back. Another spirit guide by the name Pacer has brought the young man back to just outside the vehicle. Pacer has hold of him by the arm to be sure he doesn't get scared off again and asked him to calm down.

Robert: We are all here for you.

Antoinette: The spirit guides are trying to lighten up the situation but the young man isn't having it because he's a very sad ghost. He's staying here at the house to be with his family.

Young Man: (now talking for himself again) Now I understand what I'm supposed to do. I'm just really frightened.

Robert: Everyone here around you wants to help you transition.

Young Man: So, where did you come from man? How did you know about me?

Edited to maintain anonymity.

Robert: There is a person who expressed to me that he is very concerned about you. And, off the record *(reveals the name of the person to the young man).*

Young Man: Oh! Okay. We weren't best friends.

Robert: That's true. But he was saddened with your passing and felt a concern for you.

Young Man: As were my group of close friends.

Robert: This friend knows what we do and how we are able to help people like you so you won't get stuck. He asked us to check to see if you might have gotten stuck in case you missed your opportunity.

Young Man: But now, the opening I first saw has shut down. Because I have this opportunity to speak, if I could leave you with a message maybe you could help guys my age (early twenties) or younger.

Robert: What would you tell them?

Young Man: Are you on tv?

Robert: No. But we are filming this.

Young Man: From my perspective I would say don't try

anything (substances). Don't experiment with anything. You know, I have smoked pot during my lifetime. I drank a little. But I want my message to be clear. Don't try anything. Keep it straight all the way. And, love your family because they have your back no matter what. That's all I can say.

Robert: And, you will be able to come back and check in on your family too.

Young Man: Yeah. I'm just a little scared to go.

Robert: We want to make the transition for you very easy. Pacer and Lane are incredible spirit guides.

Young Man: Yeah. Pacer was trying to tickle me before but it's not working.

Robert: We all just want to help ease your pain.

Young Man: I'm not feeling a lot of pain. What I'm feeling is about my mom. I feel like she's making me stay here. I feel like I need to hold her. And I did. And she knows I did.

Robert: I don't know if we could ever get a message about this session to your family because they don't appear to understand these things.

Young Man: Probably not. They'd probably take it as weird.

Robert: So we're doing our best to help you.

Young Man: (nods) And, I'm going! *pause* So, I have a female family member that's calling me. I don't know who she is yet but I'm going. Good bye.

Robert: Goodbye.

Note: The spirit of the twenty year old young man whose life was recently cut short (in the latter part of 2018) departs and successfully transitions.

Spirit Guide Lane: He's gone. He's transitioned to where he needed to go.

Robert: Please describe Pacer for our readers.

Spirit Guide Lane: Pacer was a 32 year-old man when he passed away about two years ago. He had resided in a beach community here locally in San Diego California. He is a new spirit guide who helps us. There is no 'free-lancing here'. Everyone here has a job to do. We send him to where his skills are needed. His job is to go to different homes and gather ghosts and moving (transitioning) them or blocking them from getting inside people's residences. He has to 'earn his wings' so-to-speak. Once he does, we'll let him talk to you.

Additionally, I would like to add my own message here. If you can all help to educate the young people about the dangers of experimenting with drugs. For instance, speak at schools about the Opioid addiction crisis. And, teach about spirituality and what really goes on here in the spirit world in regards to life after death because this poor guy (the young man) he was a mess. He had no idea about transitioning. But, he's okay now. He was a little shocked at first but he's all-right now.

So, in conclusion, we really helped this young man cross-over and he in turn is helping us by getting the word out that he is against drugs.

Robert: We've accomplished our goal here today. Now I'm going to bring Antoinette out of trance. And, we hope that we've helped you understand another facet of what is really happening around us in the spirit realm.

Robert brings Antoinette out of trance. She has become aware of other ghosts in the vicinity and begins to describe what she observed.

Antoinette: There was a female ghost near here. I don't know about the boyfriend (could be husband) but she died as a result of being on a motorcycle with him near here when they wrecked. She also crossed over with the young man. There are a lot of other ghosts around here that were trying to talk to us but it's just not their turn.

As a result of this case Robert and Antoinette have uncovered a new layer in the Opioid crisis.

As born out in this case, even experimenting with drugs can have unforeseen, dire and far reaching consequences.

As a result of the toxic effects of the substance, the person is often disoriented and disconnected from this life and their new place in the afterlife. They inhabit a void in between worlds in an unnatural state of being. Therefore, we need to add the issue of getting lost in transition, in other words, *ghosting* onto the list of potential drug side-effects.

Additionally we can chose to follow the sentiment expressed by the young man and the spirit guides in this case to infuse the efforts of those who campaign against drug abuse with our personal and financial support to keep others from falling victim to getting lost in transition.

All of the case files presented thus far have portrayed individuals passing on, ghosting, *Attaching,* and in most cases, being cleared by Robert and his team. However, An abrupt sudden death, as the result of accident or even murder of several people related to a common incident can result in ghosting. The following session is one example of how this could happen.

Out of ignorance, instead of a person here or there passing over in a disoriented state or with unfinished business, people are being sent over in masse. The upcoming Case File has been selected so that readers can begin to imagine our world in a new way that is inclusive of the spirit realm. For we exist in a world where we influence them and they in turn, affect us.

However, the actions of living human beings on each other have ripple effects into the spirit realms long after they take place.

Unfortunately, as will be seen in the next case, it is not just in war that mass loss of life happens. The United States was not at war when assailants surprised us with a terrorist attack in 2001 on the World Trade Center in New York. Here's is an account of what happened.

"On the morning of September 11, 2001, Al-Qaeda-affiliated hijackers flew two Boeing jets into the complex, one into each tower, in a coordinated act of terrorism. After burning for 56 minutes, the South Tower (2) collapsed, followed a half-hour later by the North Tower (1). The attacks on the World Trade Center killed 2,753 people. Falling debris from the towers, combined with fires that the debris initiated in several surrounding buildings, led to the partial or complete collapse of all the other buildings in the complex and caused catastrophic damage to ten other large structures in the surrounding area (including the World Financial Center). The process of cleaning up and recovery at the World Trade Center site took eight months."[5]

---

[5] Source: Wikipedia https://en.wikipedia.org/wiki/September_11_attacks October 12, 2016.

CASE FILE: In a State of Shock

Recognizing the September 11 attacks likely resulted in a ghosting situation, Robert and the team's Necormancer at the time Sam, checked in on the situation via the spiritual plane. Robert Major writes:

> Through Sam, we were able to make a spiritual connection to the area. The Spirit Guides described the people or 'souls' in shock, their clothes in shreds and bodies in tatters. Many of the victim's sat upon the rubble which existed in the same state as ours but on a kind of alternate reality which exists as a type of mirror image but on a different dimension. Appearing most like a reflection of our reality, it looks the same except those that are ghosting reside in that realm. We, the living however, do not appear there.
>
> In the weeks and months that followed, the information released by investigators and authorities was communicated to one ghost who seemed to be looking out for the others. He acted as their liaison to Sam and me. As they began to understand the situation, they began to resolve themselves to their place in it. After several months of regular communication, those that were ghosting all agreed to move on. When they did so, their confusion cleared, they could perceive the guides that had been there all along and transitioned."

When we consider that our behavior here on earth has effects beyond our physical senses and into the spirit realm we can begin to realize how this kind of destruction of life has repercussions. Despite the internalized nature of 'good' or 'bad' intentions on the part of people throughout the globe, some choices have the unintended side effect of eradicating people from this plane only to cause them to get stuck and ghost in the process. In fact, we humans are causing it on a massive scale globally from acts of terrorism, weapons of mass destruction, genocide, and wars.

If we look only at the observable, these terrorists are guilty of horrendous crimes. But if left unchecked, are they now equally dangerous ghosts?

Or, perhaps, the terrorists themselves were *Attached* at the time they piloted the planes into the twin towers. When something so shockingly devastating takes place, one can only wonder, could an *Attachment* type cycle have anything to do with extremist type incidents? It is disturbing to consider a possible link between ghosts, their influence, and devastating events that make the headlines every day but it does happen.

Because people in general are unaware of the nature of ghosts and their ability to influence the living we are unknowingly endangering ourselves and future generations by increasing the potential for people to get lost in transition in these horrific mass death incidents. It is these lost souls, along with those martyr's who died and may choose to ghost as a perceived means to an ends, that unwittingly end up ghosting. Sometimes they go on to disrupt people's lives. When they do, Robert and his team are actively doing their best to deal with the problem.

In this next case we get a perspective into how even spirits of people that have crossed over successfully are interested in helping lost souls. But, they face obstacles too.

CASE FILE: A Father's Concern for His Son

The following account is from Robert Major's case file archives which took place on Memorial Day, 2018 at the Fort Rosecrans National Cemetery.

Robert recounts: We were invited by Videographer Debra to search for ghosts to communicate with and help them cross over to the other side. Our Team had no prior knowledge of the location. Debra selected the Fort Rosecrans National Cemetery.

Upon arriving we find no one else at the cemetery. We proceed by asking our ghost sensing tech assistant if he can pick up on any spirits in the vicinity who might have an interest in what we are doing. He tells us that he already feels as if there is stuff starting to happen. He picks up upon an emotional reaction which conveys that "we don't get very many visitors."

I invite the spirits in the area to come and meet us. I reassure that each and every one that wants to cross over today can come and talk to us and we will help free them so that they can transition.

Antoinette goes into hypnotic trance and immediately begins to interact with a spirit. She conveys to us that: "There is a man here. He says hello and introduces himself as Thomas Gast.[6]

---

[6] Note: Spelling is not always exact. Sometimes names do not come through

Robert's team is making strides in obtaining names and dates from the spirit realm but sometimes names come through phonetically. In this case, Antoinette conveyed the last name as Gast instead of Gatch. However, there was enough supporting information that led post session research to conclude that his last name was Gatch.

He says he was born in the 1800s. He says that he was in both World War I and World War II and an Admiral. However, Thomas' concern is in regards to his son. He had a son, and his son has passed. Admiral Gatch was not ghosting. However, he was aware, and therefore deeply concerned, that his son had been ghosting since his death in 1974.

Often the person trapped in the ghosting state does not recognize the offer of guidance or does not trust it and may decide to ignore it. However, because Senior Gatch was connected to the communication, Antoinette was able to make contact with Thomas Gatch Jr. Junior Gatch conveyed information to Antoinette who then conveyed it to the group. She explained that it appeared to her that he made his own balloon. He went on a flying expedition in it. He's saying he went down on land. He didn't die on the day he crashed. But instead, he says, it took a couple of days.

Antoinette communicates to Thomas Gatch Jr. that his father is also in communication with her and desires that he will use this opportunity to transition now. Antoinette's spirit guide assists with the transition. Admiral Gatch

the 'medium' phonetically

53

acknowledges his awareness of the transition and expresses his gratitude to the team. They close the meeting by bidding each other farewell.

Beyond this case, Robert and the team proceed to free and transition nearly 60 souls. This means that there are that many fewer ghosts who could potentially haunt, disrupt, influence, or attach to living human beings.

The Ghost Removers know from experience communicating into spirit realms that relatives who predecease us watch over us. This is not to say they are earthbound, rather that they are in a spiritual realm that allows them to check in on us from time to time.

The same is true in this case. Since Admiral Gatch was watching over his son while he was alive he knew that when he died, he failed to make the transition. However, because they are in different realms, they were not able to communicate with each other. Their ability to affect one another is severely limited, if it can occur at all.

In the case of Admiral Gatch, he was aware of his son's failure to transition, but was helpless to do anything about it. Therefore, when Robert and his team showed up at the cemetery he seized on the opportunity to try to reach his son. This predicament could have continued indefinitely.

After returning home, Videographer Debra performed an internet search to see if she could locate concrete information that could substantiate what she witnessed that day. This is what she found.

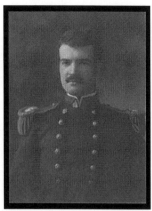

Thomas Leigh Gatch as a young Naval officer[7]

US Navy Vice Admiral Gatch was born August 9, 1981 in Salem, Oregon and died at age 63 on December 16, 1954 in San Diego, CA. He is buried at the Fort Rosecrans National Cemetery. His years of military service was from 1912 to 1947 during which he held the command of Judge Advocate General, Atlantic Fleet service force, USS South Dakota. He served in both World War I and World War II as well as in the Battle of the Santa Cruz Islands. He was awarded two Navy Cross and a Purple Heart.

---

[7] Source: https://en.wikipedia.org/wiki/Thomas_Leigh_Gatch

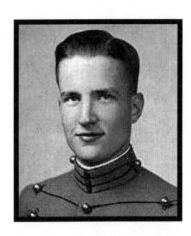

Thomas Leigh Gatch, Jr.

An internet search for Admiral Gatch's son confirmed that Thomas Leigh Gatch, Jr. was lost in a balloon over the Atlantic. He was last sighted February 21, 1974 about 1,000 miles west of the Canary Islands. He was 48 at the time.[8]

In this case, Admiral Gatch kept a watchful eye over his son who failed to transition after his death. From this and other cases, Robert and his team have come to understand the loved ones watch over each other in this life as well as the next.

In the same manner, the concept of leaving no man behind that is used by those in military in regards to battle or service can be applicable in regards to ghosts too. The concept of the Latin phrase nemo resideo, or "leave no one behind," is almost as old as warfare itself.

---

[8] Source: http://www.west-point.org/users/usma1946/15885/

The United States has always held to the sacred rule that we don't leave our men or women in uniform behind. Some wonder why is it worth risking the lives of more soldiers just to bring one lone man or woman in uniform home? To others, the ends justifies the means.

Certainly, not all ghosts lost their lives as a result of military service, but many have. Any one of us has the potential to become lost in transition. Therefore, it stands to reason, that each of us could also become a troublesome spirit to living human beings. Given the number of people that die every day on the planet, one can see how widespread the problem likely is. And, it could be affecting each and every one of us in one way or another.

Ghosts exist in a space between our world and the next. In essence, they are trapped there. Yet, little thought is given to whether or not we can help them. It is important to consider how we can work hand-in-hand with the spirit realm to guide spirits of our lost brethren safely to their next home so that they are not left behind..

The case of Admiral Gatch is yet another example that the familial ties are not cut upon death. Loved ones continue to check in to assess the on the state of others. It also highlights the barriers we the living share with those in the spirit realm regarding transversing realms. Currently, only a human medium can speak to spirits of the dead on multi-dimensional levels of existence. Admiral Gatch was able to perceive that his son had died and failed to transition. However, he was unable to transverse to the another realm in order to help his son to the afterlife. Instead, he communicated his concern for Thomas Gatch Jr. to Antoinette and Robert, who, along with their spirit guides, assisted Gatch Jr. to successfully transition. Perhaps, in time, a technology will be developed that can aid in communicating with different realms.

CHAPTER 4:
EARTHBOUND SPIRITS THAT INTERACT WITH THE LIVING

No matter which version of the afterlife one ascribes to, there is the possibility of the spirit getting lost in the transition after death which results in the state of ghosting. The textbook definition of a ghost is the spirit of a dead person or animal that has not successfully transitioned to the afterlife. That is an unnatural and undesirable state of being. Ghosts can haunt particular locations, objects, or even people indefinitely.

For instance, haunted hotels are known to exist in historically populated areas throughout the world. These are places where people stayed for a time before moving on. Occasionally, tragedies occurred there. As a result, sometime in the past, one or more guests checked in but never checked out. In fact, these guests never leave. Instead, they haunt.

There are internet resources available for those who seek information about everything from finding paranormal activity in their area to haunted travel destinations. An internet search of haunted places in Southern California will result in directing you to Coronado. Coronado is a resort city on a peninsula in the San Diego Bay. Coronado is most known for the grand Victorian Hotel Del Coronado. It is one of the view surviving examples of the wooden Victorian architectural genre. It is the second largest wooden structure in the United States and is a national historic landmark.

When it opened in 1888 it was the largest resort hotel in the world. It has hosted royalty, presidents, and celebrities through the years. For instance, the Prince of Wales and Wallace Simpson were hotel guests. As were 16 presidents from John F. Kennedy to Barack Obama. From the filming of the movie *Some Like It Hot* with Marilyn Monroe to Oprah Winfrey the celebrity and notables guest list reads like a *Who's Who* of the time period.

However, this is where our story is about to take a different turn. Hotel guest Kate Morgan's suicide at the Hotel Del Coronado in November of 1892 generated widespread publicity throughout the state of California. Because little was known about Kate's identity the press began to refer to her as *The Beautiful Stranger.*

In 2002 the Hotel del Coronado Heritage Department published a book entitled *Beautiful Stranger: The Ghost of Kate Morgan and the Hotel Del Coronado.* The official account of

Kate Morgan's 1892 visit to the Hotel del Coronado and why it is believed that she haunts today, as well as an accurate account of her mysterious life and death.

On the book cover, Kate is depicted as she has been described by a hotel guest who sketched her in elegant Victorian attire.

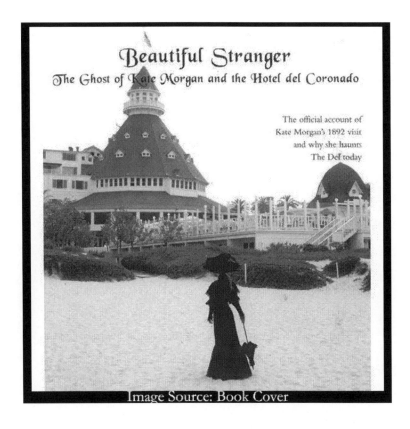

Beautiful Stranger
The Ghost of Kate Morgan and the Hotel del Coronado

The official account of
Kate Morgan's 1892 visit
and why she haunts
The Del today

Image Source: Book Cover

The account in the book revealed that Kate had checked into the hotel under an assumed name the public interest only increased. *Who was the beautiful stranger? Where had she* come from? *Why did she travel to the Hotel Del Coronado? And, why had she taken her own life?*

What is important for the Ghost Removers is why Kate Morgan is reputed to be ghosting the Hotel Del. Following a hunch that there is more to the story, Robert and Antoinette decided to investigate the haunting further.

CASE FILE: *The Haunted Hotel*
This is what happened in the *The Ghost Remover Chronicle Case of the Haunted Hotel (GRC Case #0110).*

Hypnotherapist Robert and Trance-Channel Antoinette went to the public beach access area adjacent to the hotel in early 2019. Here is a transcription of the recording.

Robert: It is rumored that this place is heavily haunted. And we're here today to visit and find out what's really going on. I'm a hypnotherapist, and Antoinette will enter a hypnotic trance and she will be able to communicate with them and tell us their story.

Antoinette: I'm just about to go into trance with my hypnotherapist Robert so we can communicate with ghosts. Here we go!

Antoinette enters into trance and her spirit guide Lane communicates through her. He is going to detail ghosts that are in the area. And, he is there to make sure that communication between Antoinette and ghosts is clear.

Lane: I don't have Kate here. I have the spirit of another lady who drowned here. She's right here to my left. Her name is Isadore. She is a woman who drowned here.

Robert. How long ago?

Lane: 1904.

Robert: Has she been the one ghosting all this time?

Lane: Yes. And, Kate Morgan is on the premises too. Isadore and Kate do not get along. Now, I'll step out and let the spirits communicate through Antoinette.

Antoinette: Isadore is here. She was beautiful and attired in a Victorian style look including what looks like a corset. She's telling me that she was a stage actress in theater. She's saying that she was pretty famous for her looks. She's telling me that she drowned here. But not because she couldn't swim. She drowned because she had an illness in the area of her upper chest and is clutching that area. I think the water may have shocked her but I don't know for sure. I can't really read that.

Robert: How old would she be?

Antoinette: When she died? Hold on . . . Isadore is saying

that she can hear you Robert. She's showing me 38 years old. Still very young.

Robert: Do you frequent the hotel all the time?

Isadore: (now speaking as herself) Yes, I'm staying here now. I'm on the third floor. Kate is on the same floor but I don't listen to her. There is another ghost here to. Three females (Isadore, Kate, and Sonya) and one male named Benjamin who died around 1890. Benjamin and I get along. Sonya is a recluse. However, Kate is a sad ghost. I'm not so sad. I'm a socialite and I love all the different people here. I can go moving in and out of walls as well as people.

Benjamin and I frequent the beach and pretend to feel the water because living people can feel it but we can't. We ghosts still have emotions but we don't have the physical sense of touch so we cannot feel things. However, by being half-in Antoinette's body at this time, I can feel your arm on her body and it feels good to experience the sensation of touch again.

Robert: Which ghost carries the parasol?

Isadore: I am the person depicted as carrying the parasol. I'm the lady pictured on the beach and the one portrayed in the historical writings. That's me!

Robert: Okay then, we're starting to figure this out. You

(Isadore) and Kate are two different ghosts. Why are you ghosting Isadore?

Isadore: I'm ghosting because I don't want to cross over. I'm living here in this manner. I will cross-over when I feel like it but I'm not ready yet.

On the other hand, Kate might want to transition. Kate is a sad ghost. She doesn't leave her room. She stays in there and causes trouble. Kate makes noises, jiggles things trying to be scary, moans a lot, slamming things, and has tantrums.

Antoinette: Kate is a poltergeist.

Isadore's message to the living is to: Love life and people while you are alive because you never know how long your life will be.

Robert: Is there a way we can help you Isadore?

Isadore: No. I'm not looking for help. *Pauses for a few moments in silence.* I'm leaving now.

Note: As Isadore departs Antoinette's body, Antoinette's body falls forward for a second. Robert puts his hand on her back in order to hold her upright until Antoinette re-orients herself fully back into her own body.

Antoinette: She's gone.

Robert brings Antoinette out of hypnotic trance.

Antoinette: When I'm under trance and I step aside for another spirit, in this case Isadore, she was half-in and half-out and letting me stay to listen because she wasn't sure she wanted to come all the way in, because she hadn't done that before. At the end of our session today, Isadore stepped out. This process also occurs when my spirit guide Lane comes in. He comes in, sometimes half so I can hear everything that is going on then he steps out.

What I remember most about Isadore from where I was during the conversation was that she was very beautiful and a very talented stage actress. I was shown a replay of her plays during which she sang, danced, and was so happy doing that. That's what impressed me most about Isadore.

Robert: What we really came here for today was to visit with Kate. But that did not happen . Instead we found out that there are four ghosts present here. Kate is one of them. She has poltergeist capabilities. According to Isadore, Kate is a sad ghost who has secluded herself in her room on the third floor. The ghost that has been seen and described out and about the Hotel Del Coronoado grounds and on the beach is Isadore.

Next, Robert checks the internet on his phone. This is what he finds.

Robert: This is the information we just found. In 1904 Hotel Del Coronado introduced the first electricity. Also in 1904, Actress Isadore Rush drowned. That's all the research I can do from here. I'll return home and do some additional research on Isadore Rush to find out the story behind her.

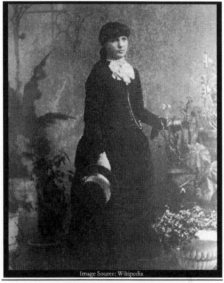

Kate Morgan

From Wikipedia on Kate Morgan was born Kate Farmer in Fremont Iowa around 1864. She has also been known as Lottie Bernard.

Kate's mother died in the summer of 1865 when Kate was only a year old. At the age of two she was sent to live with her maternal grandfather Joe Chandler. In December of 1885 Kate married Thomas Morgan. They had one child, a boy, born in October of 1886. He survived only two days.

Around 1890 Kate is reported to have left her husband for Albert Alan. Kate's trail picks up again in Southern California in the Los Angeles area when she is working for the Grant family as a house maid. Kate told coworkers that she was married to a gambler. From this statement her husband Tom Morgan was assumed to be the gambler in question. But in fact, he was a rural mail carrier in Nebraska at the time of Kate's death.

Housekeeper Kate checked into the Hotel Del Coronado room 302 under the name of Lottie Bernard on Thanksgiving Day of 1892.

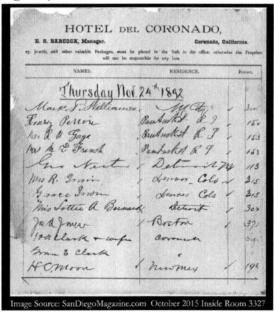

Image Source: SanDiegoMagazine.com October 2015 Inside Room 3327

Kate spent five days meandering through the Del alone. Some claim that she was waiting for her husband. Others say that Kate was anticipating a lover's arrival.

68

At the time of her death, Kate was found dead on the exterior staircase of the Hotel Del Coronado leading to the beach. Kate's death was determined to be a suicide by a gunshot wound to her head. There is much speculation surrounding possible motives for her action. But no clear evidence exists that would explain why Kate would take her own life.

The state of being a poltergeist can be the result of sadness or even anger. If Kate experienced tragedy of a different nature, it might explain her current behavior as a ghosting poltergeist. If future communication with the Ghost Removers and Kate were to take place, it would need to occur in the room in which she resides in. By talking with Kate directly more of her story could be uncovered. Perhaps, as a result of a meeting with the Ghost Removers and their spirit guides Kate could finally find the help she needs to be at peace.

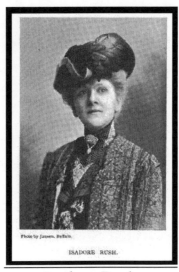

Photo by Jansen, Buffalo.

ISADORE RUSH.

Isadore Rush

A similar internet search for Isadore Rush brings her story to light. Isadore was born in 1866 in Pennsylvania. She was a stage actress who performed in vaudeville and on Broadway.

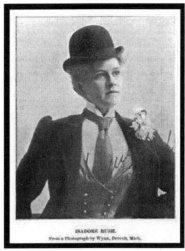

ISADORE RUSH.
From a Photograph by Wyss, Detroit, Mich.

Isadore was married to comedian Roland Reid. Previously she was married to a man named White and by him had a daughter Maude White who was a young stage actress at the time of Rush's death.

It was reported by the San Francisco Chronicle at the time that, while bathing in the surf that afternoon, Miss Isadore Rush, the well-known actress and the star of Glittering Gloria Company which was billed to appear at the Isis theater that night was caught by a mammoth breaker and swept out to sea. Several persons hastened to her assistance and she was brought ashore unconscious. Two physicians were promptly at hand and they exerted every known means to resuscitate Miss Rush. Shortly after four o'clock the actress was pronounced dead.

The sea during the past few days had been unusually high and dangerous even for the most practiced swimmer. Miss Rush had the reputation of being something of an athlete and had taken much interest in sports of all kinds. She was a fair swimmer but even the most proficient man would have had difficulty with the surf that was running that afternoon.

Commentary

There has been some confusion in the past about the ghosting activity at the Hotel Del Coronado in part because the activity was attributed to one ghost instead of two.

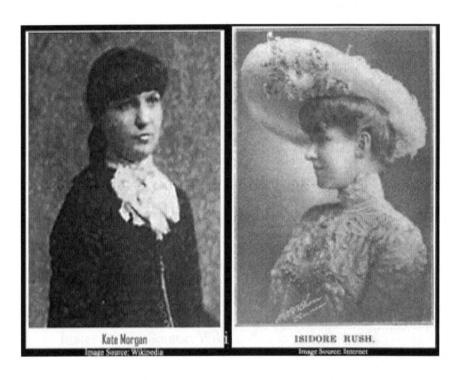

Kate Morgan
Image Source: Wikipedia

ISIDORE RUSH.
Image Source: Internet

As a result of Robert and Antoinette's exploration into this case we can look at the previous reported paranormal activity at the Hotel del Coronado with a new perspective. For example, one could look at uniquely distinct footprints in the sand for telltale signs of who might have walked there such as size and depth of the foot impressions could distinguish that there had been more than one individual who had walked there.

Instead of footprints in the sand however, each ghost leaves its own trace signature from its behavior. Kate's behavior coincides with that of a poltergeist capable of manipulating the physical world. Whereas in comparison Isadore's behavior is more subtle. Isadore's appearance is more like what observer's have described as Victorian. Isadore moves about the hotel where Kate is described by Isadore as staying in her room. Therefore we are observing that there is more than one ghost responsible for the paranormal activity at the Hotel Del Coronado. Kate and Isadore are two of them.

Robert and Antoinette would like the opportunity to try and help Kat Morgan. But if a future communication with Kate were to occur it would need to take place in the room she haunts. For now however, Robert and Antoinette are satisfied that they have uncovered a new layer of information regarding the mystery of the 'beautiful stranger' who haunts the hotel.

As we have discovered, to perform an internet search of haunted places in Southern California will result in directing you to Coronado and to the Hotel del Coronado. There are internet resources available for people who seek information about things like haunted places nearby including haunted hotels. Haunted hotels are known to exist in historically populated areas throughout the world. There are places where people stayed for a time before moving on. Occasionally tragedies occurred there. As a result, sometime in the past one or more guests checked in but never checked out. In fact, these guests never leave. Instead, they haunt.

The Ghost Remover team includes a core group of spirit guides and helpers. A few of them specifically have the role of transitioning wayward spirits of the dead. In the end, Spirit helpers hand off the wayward spirits to the spirit guide that has been waiting all along to help them move on to the afterlife. In time, perhaps they can assist Kate Morgan towards a successful transition.

CHAPTER 5:
GHOSTING TO *ATTACHMENT*

Ghost stories abound in both oral and written accounts. The living have told and retold versions of lost souls who haunt from phantom armies, ghost trains, phantom ships and even ghost animals. This book is not about earthbound entities in general but only those that *Attach*.

Most people are familiar with the terms ghosts and haunting. However, *Attachments* is likely altogether new. There is a distinction between ghosting, haunting and *Attachments*. A ghost is the spirit of someone lost in transition between this life and the next. A haunting is the act of the ghost to visit habitually or appear frequently as a spirit to haunt a location or a person. Whereas *Attachments* are spirits that engage in a parasitic relationship with a living person. Effects can range from mild-to-severe.

A mild *Attachment* might have the effect of recurring persistently to the consciousness of a person and remaining in their thoughts and memories. A moderate *Attachment* might influence a person's behavior. A severe *Attachment* can take over a person completely and possess them for a short or long period of time.

In other words, ghosts act out all the time and in different ways as in the next case involving remote viewing. Remote viewing is clairvoyant practice of seeking impressions about a distant or unseen person, place, or object using subjective means such as extrasensory perception (ESP) or "sensing with mind." Typically a remote viewer gets information that is hidden from physical view and separated at some distance. While remote viewing became well known to the public in the 1970's, it has actually been around for a very long time.

SESSION: Encounter on a Coastal Boardwalk
One afternoon on a busy coastal boardwalk in Pacific Beach, California, Remote Viewer and Ghost Remover Marcos demonstrated his ability to use remote viewing to an agent who wanted to film the session to create a 'Sizzle'. A Sizzle is a two or three minute promotional video which talent agents submit to television production companies. After watching the video of the session that day, here is what I observed.

> While in hypnotic trance, facing away and perpendicular to the boardwalk, Marcos was able to continually describe people who passed by behind him that he could not visually see because of his positioning. In some instances he described their clothes, in other cases he gave an account of facial features. He went on to identify who amongst them were *Attached* along with the history of their *Attachment* and the influence it was having on the human host.
>
> Shortly into the video, a young man wearing a book

type back pack, had passed behind Marcos. The passerby was heading South on the boardwalk. Marcos never turned around to look at this passerby directly, but here's what happened next. Marcos remotely engaged the *Attachment* who resided on the young man who was by then, about a hundred feet away. The *Attachment* then acted out and took over the fellow. As it did so, he turned around and headed towards Marcos. Robert placed himself between the two physically to protect Marcos should the entity attack.

The interaction between Marcos and the fellow was invisible to any onlooker because it was taking place remotely and on the level the ghost resided upon which was out of the range of living human beings to see.

The *Attachments* took over the fellow's body and was animating it. In other words, the three ghosts fully possessed the young man's body and was in complete control of it. *They* came closer and stopped about fifty feet short of Marcos where *they* remained on the grassy knoll adjacent to the opposite side of the sidewalk from Marcos.

As Marcos communicated with the *Attachments, they* responded through the fellow. *They* yelled, swore and threatened Marcos. One of the *Attachments* exclaimed, 'We're not going anywhere!' At one point, *they* got down on *their* hands and knees and repeatedly pounded his fist on the ground. For all intents and purposes it appears the fellow was, by himself acting crazy for no apparent reason. But to those who are aware of *Attachments,* there was an explanation for what transpired that day.

After Marcos severed the communication with the *Attachments,* the entities retreated back to where it was before the engagement. The young man, now back in control of his body, stood up and walked away appearing to be like any other normal person walking down the boardwalk that day.

Now, you might ask, "What creates vulnerability to *Attachments?*" The answer is weakness. One effect of traumatic events in your life, whether they are physical, mental or emotional is that they can create weakness in your energetic self also known as the Subtle Body, leaving you vulnerable to being *Attached.* Many of the Case Files recounted in this book provide different examples of what this can be like.

As has been mentioned previously, ghosts are spirits that have lived on earth but remain earthbound. A sudden death, as in combat, can leave a soul dazed and confused. Therefore, military personnel that have been in combat are particularly susceptible to ghosting situations. Their similar experiences and close proximity to the dead and dying can increase the vulnerability for and proximity to ghosts leading to *Attachment* incidents.

There are many individual accounts of experiences in the military that lead to lingering distress. The symptoms may appear as Post Traumatic Stress Disorder (PTSD). Some of these people have found their way or been referred to the Ghost Removers for help, especially when they do not find relief through conventional means. However, many military clients don't want anyone else to know that they were cleared of an *Attachment*. Due to their training and military 'code of conduct' they are very uncomfortable about this and as a result, remain silent.

Though *not* an actual case file, the following scenario contains elements that are typical of *Attachment* situations. This account was selected because it concisely depicts some of the language typically heard in cases involving the presence of an *Attachment*. The description is an account of a U.S. soldier's experience during WWII which haunted him until his death.

"We could no longer engage the enemy from a safe distance. My unit was advancing into the village. I, along with the other men, made our way forward dodging bullets as we sprinted to the next rubble or debris that could shield us. I couldn't see the enemy. Their shots rang out from war-torn buildings ravaged from previous bombing raids. I was hidden behind the remains of a corner of a building. After a few moments, I glanced over what remained of the front wall. My eyes met those of an enemy soldier who was squatting down in the shadow of the room in the opposite corner to where I was positioned. I quickly assessed that he was armed with only a knife. His face was dirty and his uniform in tatters. He appeared to be about my age, late teens, maybe twenty. After the brief hesitation when our eyes locked, he sprung to his feet wielding the knife to attack me. In response, I shot him. He was the first man I'd ever shot at point blank range. I jumped the wall and walked the few steps to where he lay on the ground. He looked up into my eyes as his body heaved its last breath. This young man was a stranger to me. But I still had to shoot him.

Our assault continued on long into the night. The incident didn't bother me the first night. I was so tired I slept from exhaustion. But the second night I woke up crying because that soldier's face was there. He was in my dreams. I was haunted by the image of his face and his eyes that seemed to lock on mine even though my eyes were closed. To this day I wake up many nights and I still see him in my dreams. I don't know how to get him off my mind."

In cases where someone is haunted by a person or a memory, pay attention to the language used for it holds the key to what is really happening. There are telling similarities in the terminology and the presence of an *Attachment*. In this situation, he states, "I don't know how to get *him* off my mind." If this case were the result of an *Attachment*, the influence would appear to be on the mild side as a haunting. An indication of a more serious case would be if the surviving soldier was periodically acting *out of character*. Often the other *character traits* are the result of the influencing or haunting personality rather than those of the host. The behavior displayed when the *Attachment* has taken over and possessed the host offers indicators as to *who* the *Attachment* was when he or she was alive, before they were ghosting. Those personality traits often carry over with them and are distinctly different from the host.

In addition to physical, mental and emotional trauma which is done to you or in other ways, out of your control, there is another way to create vulnerability to *Attachments*. That is to create weakness in yourself. This can happen with substance abuse.

In the not too distant past, liquor store signs that read "Beer, Wine & *Spirits*" were commonplace. There are several theories as to why liquor is called *Spirits*. Technically, they are differentiated from beer and wine by a distilling process which is believed to contain the essence of the ingredients.

In a case where any substance is abused, your body may become too toxic for your spirit and it can actually leave. As your spirit *passes-out* of your body, you leave an access point for a ghosting entity to *Attach*. And very often, considering that like attracts like, the type of spirit that wants to *Attach* can be a toxic one. In the case of alcohol, ghosts that were alcoholic while alive are attracted to the alcohol poisoned body like a patron to a bar. Once it latches on, from that point forward the alcoholic ghost *Attached* to the living human being drives the person to drink more because *they* want the experience of inebriation. The same process occurs with drugs. So, this is where the problems begin and in the future, compounds for the victim of the *Attachment* who has unwittingly placed themselves in jeopardy.

Whether stemming from physical, mental, emotional trauma or self-imposed vulnerability, ghosts can read you just like a diagnostic imaging machine and determine your weakness. The reason that ghosts have that ability is because they perceive on a realm that is nearer to the Subtle Body. On that level, the living appear more like their elements of light, color, and pattern.

One big motivator for these spirits to *Attach* is the opportunity to experience life again. Some are content with only a fragment of a life while others want more. Then there are those who have their own reasons for *Attaching* such as supporting a cause they were part of while alive.

These entities don't care if you are good or bad. They don't differentiate between who is young or old, only who is a target. As prey to dark spirits, previous trauma victims are often re-victimized because the weakness in their Subtle Body remains untreated. This is not to say that the same issue repeatedly occurs to the person. Sometimes the problems are in the same vein, other times it is more a case of bad things that keep happening seemingly without any root cause.

If you think an *Attachment* could not influence or *Attach* to someone you know . . . even to YOU . . . think again. Ordinary people do get *Attached*. Unfortunately for some *Attachment* victims, it is a case of being perceived as vulnerable while merely in the wrong place at the wrong time.

CASE FILE: Ghosts Attack
Recounted by Robert:

> "It started late one night after my sister Antoinette had picked up her two nieces, Chantelle and Michelle, at a nearby Vons supermarket and brought them home to stay the night. She said that

Michelle had gotten into an argument with her stepmom earlier that evening and asked to stay with her. Antoinette told me there were strange noises in the house and that she felt dark spirits had entered. I told her I would come over to check it out. By the time I got there everything was quiet. They had told the ghosts I was coming and they had better leave.

I put Michelle into a trance to calm her. While hypnotized, Michelle said she could see and hear the ghosts and they hadn't cleared out after all. She started telling me what the ghosts were saying. They wanted her to commit suicide and be part of their group. Then I proceeded to put my sister Antoinette in trance so we could get some help from our spirit guides from the other side. Right as Antoinette entered trance she started gasping for air." "We will just see how good you are!" this creepy voice yelled out. She was being choked. This went on for about ten seconds before our spirit guide we call Lane, arrived and stopped the attack.

It took a few moments for my sister to revive. I could see red hand prints around her neck. This was the most radical we had encountered so far while doing this type of work. Fortunately Lane was quick to restrain the ghost and sent him on to the other side. He then proceeded to do the same with the rest.

Afterwards, Lane told us that the ghost who was the leader was named Steve. He had committed suicide just like the other five had. They wanted to drive Michelle to suicide so she could be part of

Steve's entourage. The ghosts were there in the Vons parking lot loitering about when they picked up Michelle's emotional state following the argument earlier that evening with her mother which resulted in her leaving the house and go to Vons.

It was while Michelle was at Vons that they *Attached* to Michelle who was then picked up by Antoinette and taken to her house. From Lane we learned that Steve and the others were hoping to send Michelle over the edge emotionally that night. They intended to augment and amplify her already despondent emotional state and drive her to suicide so that Michelle could join them where they were. Luckily for her, we were able to intervene and stop them."

For another perspective on this same case, here is Michelle's account of that evening as she relayed it to Robert.

Okay, so what I remember is Antoinette came and picked me and Chantelle up from Vons cause I got into a fight with my stepmother. Antoinette was about to go to bed when she said she saw a cloud type thing. Then we heard footsteps going upstairs but there was no one else at home. We went outside for a cigarette and when we walked back in her son Eric's shoe flew across the floor seemingly by itself. Chy Chy, Antoinette's dog would not leave my side. That's when Antoinette called you and the three of us started telling it that you were coming to help us. Things immediately got quiet. When I talked to the spirits, we all could hear them talking in low angry unintelligible voices. There was more than one talking but we couldn't understand what they were saying. Then everyone tried talking to them but they would not respond. They would only talk to me!"

"The whole time Chy Chy would not leave my side and we all knew that wasn't normal. Eric, now in the room too, even grabbed his camera and actually got footage of the apparition. When you (Robert) finally got there you decided to put me under trance with Antoinette because they were only answering me. Come to find out there were six males *Attached* to me around my neck! They had a plan to have me commit suicide before it was morning; they wanted me to be the seventh person. Then, you removed them from me."

"I still can hear the demonic voice that came through Antoinette. And, when me and Chantelle were talking about what happened I can actually remember when they *Attached* to me. While we were waiting for Antoinette to come pick us up Chantelle told me a handicapped male walked by us and I made a very rude comment. That was very strange for me to do something like that. And I remember on the back of his shirt had my name (Michelle) on it! I remember at that moment feeling anger, hate, jealousy, and every bad emotion a human could feel!!! At the time, I didn't understand what was happening to me."

"By sharing my experience with Robert I'm glad my story will finally be able to reach other people and hopefully some of them may realize what can happen. I am very proud of you and what you have accomplished and the people you have helped! I read about the lady you helped that had an *Attachment* since she was two years old. That's insane! But if anybody understands it's me!!"

These lost spirits need help moving on and the Ghost Remover team has developed a method to do just that. It is the unique combination of trance work, mediumship and *voluntary* possession channeling combined with teams from the spirit world and the physical world working together to clear the victim and help the lost soul find its way. The Ghost Removers make no judgment about where the *Attachments* go after they are removed. They trust the spirit guides to act in the highest and best interests of those involved.

As a result of the guidance from spirit helpers, the Ghost Remover process has evolved over the years to become very adept in managing a wide variety of circumstances. What has emerged is a Ghost Remover process that is a hybrid of both spiritual thinking and modern analysis. In contrast to the traditional methods of *deliverance* and *exorcism designed to remove demons*, the Ghost Remover process includes a team of people including hypnotist, psychic team, and spirit guides. Together they identify who is *Attached*, remove the *Attachment*, and send it on to its next stage of evolution in the afterlife. Then they repair the Subtle Body opening that allowed the *Attachment(s)* to enter in the first place. The process is an especially unique method. Based upon client feedback, their process is effective.

In the following chapters we will explore what that looks like through more actual case files and team experiences in an effort to provide a real sense of the true nature of the *Attachment* dilemma.

CHAPTER 6:
THE NATURE OF
MILDLY SEVERE
ATTACHMENTS

Since the time of their first removal, the Ghost Remover team has worked on thousands of cases. During that time they have been able to observe certain patterns and elements that are indicators of possible *Attachments*. Situations that are likely ghost related can happen on many levels of severity.

Therefore, having an *Attachment* can look very different on different people. The effects are also specific to the individual based on the ghost spirit that *Attached*, their motives and personality. As we have seen in cases presented thus far, there is an element of the law of attraction at work. In other words, "like attracts like", which can compound a person's problems and exacerbate emotions. The following cases are examples of this diversity.

CASE FILE: Shopaholic
Julia is a strikingly beautiful and fashionable woman about fifty years of age. Born in the 1950's into a large family, her parents were poor and her family struggled with the effects

of living with an alcoholic father. Despite the problems of her youth she has class, style, and the rare ability to comfortably engage with almost anyone. However, she struggled with a compulsion to over shop.

Julia was referred by a mutual friend to Robert. The following is her account of what happened.

> I was confiding to my girlfriend that I felt my current relationship problems had a lot to do with emotional struggles from my childhood. After hearing my story, she suggested that I might be *Attached*. I'd never heard of that before but I knew her well and trusted her advice. I gave her my full birth name and birthdate which she forwarded to Robert to check me for the presence of an *Attachment*. She got back to me and said that Robert had confirmed that I was indeed *Attached*.

> After making an appointment for the removal I remember experiencing a new sense of feeling very anxious and emotionally up. This persisted until the appointment itself. It was odd. I didn't know *It* was there before then but now I wasn't sure how I'd feel without *It* because *It* had seemed so much a part of me. There was a feeling of angst inside of me. I felt what can best be described as a sense of being disrupted. I now know that was what the *Attachment* was feeling, not me.

> During the appointment, while Marcos was working on me, I felt a pulling on my throat area. In the past, whenever I'd get emotional, my throat tightened up a lot. And, I remembered when I was

younger I always felt there was something in my throat. It is interesting that Marcos went right to my throat area to clear out the *Attachment*. I felt him pulling it. I felt *It* leaving but it was a struggle for sure. *It* didn't want to go. Marcos had to tug a lot to get *It* out.

Marcos went on to describe what he sensed about the nature of the *Attachment*. He told me there were actually two. One was much stronger and the other weaker. They stemmed from a couple of major incidences in my childhood. One came on around age 5 or 6 during some trauma I was experiencing at the time. There were so many back then so I didn't specifically identify which event it might have been. The other came in when I was a bit older. At age 13, I was really sick with a high fever of 105. I recall feeling like I died and came back. It was the kind of near death experience people talk about today. I distinctly remember it. I concluded that I got *Attached* then.

Marcos told me they were making me do compulsive things. They enticed me to act compulsively in general but had the most strength to cause compulsive over-shopping during times when I felt sad, lonely, neglected, or not loved. The shopping would make me feel better. It felt like an instant fix for the empty spot inside of me.

After they were removed, I immediately felt very relaxed, calm and relieved. It felt like a big brick had been taken off me. Ever since, (about four years now) I'm more in control of my own thoughts and feelings. I have more control of compulsions and emotions including my shopping and spending.

Sometimes the *Attachment* can actually seem copacetic. It is not always clear from the start what is actually going on as evidenced in this case.

CASE FILE: Lounge Singer

By all accounts Brian, a middle-aged man in his forties who worked as a mechanic, had the talent to be a big star. He'd been the lead singer for many different groups over the years but so far, he hadn't been discovered. He would be an ideal candidate to be on and discovered by a talent show. Instead, Brian seems to have become content with a weekly gig as a lounge singer.

Robert checked Brian for the presence of an *Attachment*. It turns out, Brian was *Attached*. At first it appeared as if the *Attachment* had spirit guide qualities about it because he was attracted to Brian as a result of the shared interest in singing and seemed to be supportive of that avocation. The spirit was that of a deceased lounge singer and found a common bond with Brian. They both had great talent but never hit it big professionally. In certain circumstances like Brian's, where the *Attachment* appeared to do no harm to the host, it might seem plausible to allow it to remain. In this case, *It,* having made a convincing argument to remain, was left on Brian for a time. However, it didn't take long for other side-effects of *Its* presence came to light. Allowing *It* to remain outweighed any benefit it may have offered and so was removed.

Clearing Brian of the Lounge Singer was one of the very early Ghost Remover cases. A lot has been learned since then. Some *Attachments,* as with the one on Brian, make their case, even plead to stay on their host. But the common element in every instance is that the pleadings are always self-serving. *It* wasn't pleading to stay to help Brian achieve his desire of becoming a professional singer. Being *Attached* to Brian allowed *It* to come out every week while at the lounge. *It* wanted another chance but it wasn't his time it was Brian's turn to shine. For all we know *It's* shortage of talent and star quality may have kept him back in his lifetime and held Brian back in this one too. In any case, the current protocol is to remove all *Attachments* because the risks outweigh any benefit.

The Ghost Removers have encountered many types of *Attachments* over the twenty years or so they have been doing this work. Some are mild, others are moderate-to-severe, but they have learned a great deal about the problem and have refined their process to help victims wherever they find them.

There are times when a person happens to come to their attention through unique circumstances as in the next case.

CASE FILE: The Interview
Robert recounts what happened one day when he and two of his team members are interviewed by a Los Angeles, CA area Production Company.

"I was contacted by the Vice President of a Production Company.", recalls Robert. "One of her assistants had come across our information on GhostRemover.com and had suggested us as candidates for a potential reality TV series. Antoinette, Marcos and I were very excited at the prospect of bringing the issue of *Attachments* to a much larger audience. We wanted to help a lot more people and this venue might help us do that."

"We made the short trip from San Diego to Los Angeles. Once inside the office building we were seated in a conference room where we waited about ten minutes for the V.P. to join us. Upon entering, she greeted us enthusiastically. She wasted no time before asking many different questions regarding our abilities. After sharing a few case histories with her, we offered to give a live demonstration. I put Antoinette and Marcos into hypnotic trance. I then asked Marcos if anyone present was *Attached*. He said there was. The assistant to the V.P., who had joined the meeting a few minutes late, was *Attached*. Marcos proceeded to describe the *Attachment* and what it was doing to her and her life. She confirmed the assessment. With her permission we proceeded to remove the *Attachment*."

Robert continues, "Both the V.P. and her assistant were very impressed. The V.P. inquired if there were any other employees on that floor of the office building that were *Attached*. Marcos, a gifted remote viewer, scanned the area and identified a man two offices down the hall as being *Attached*. Without ever having seen the man, Marcos described him as wearing a plaid shirt and glasses and having tattoos on his arms. Right away the V.P. said she knew who he was talking about and asked her assistant to go and bring the man into the conference room which she did."

"As he entered, we could see that he was wearing a black and red plaid shirt, black horned rim glasses and he had tattoos on both of his arms. He had no idea who we were, why we were there, or what we were doing. At the request of the V.P., he sat down. Without further ado Marcos described to the man how he'd been *Attached* during a time he was down and out and homeless a few years ago. He was quite surprised at the information being presented, especially in front of his boss. He had not shared that with anybody. Marcos went on to describe what the *Attachment* was doing to him. It was sabotaging personal relationships. It was also creating issues with his ongoing projects. One of those projects was for the OWN network. The man agreed with the assessment and was willing to go forward with the removal which we did for him."

"As it turns out, translating what we do into a format for television presented its own set of difficulties. We are still hopeful that those problems can be worked out." concludes Robert.

Attachments are spirits that are still wandering the earth. They are lost souls who may try to influence, haunt and even take over without the consent of their human host in an effort to gain some kind of control or connection to what they see as being alive, not truly recognizing that they are in fact dead. The Ghost Remover team has developed long term relationships with spirit helpers whose job it is to help these wayward spirits. That is why they have chosen the Ghost Removers as their conduit to the living. They are purely interested in helping these spirits move on.

CHAPTER 7:
THE NATURE OF
MODERATELY SEVERE
ATTACHMENTS

There are many kinds of emotional trauma. Being the victim of a crime is certainly one of the worst traumas one could experience. Ghost Remover case files are full of physically and emotionally traumatized people who have come to them for *Attachment* removals.

CASE FILE: Maria was Led by an Inner Voice to Find Me

Robert recounts, "A number of years back when we were just learning about *Attachments* and the influence they can have over people I was reminded of a peculiar incident from my sister Antoinette." She phoned me one day to tell me her sister-in-law Paulette called her to tell her about what had transpired over the past few days. Paulette said that three days prior she was in the front of her home watering the lawn. A woman got her attention. As she approached me she said, "I don't want to startle you. My name is Maria. I have a voice in my head telling me you know a man named Robert who can help me." Paulette told Antoinette that she was taken aback by the woman and her inquiry. Instead of thinking about it she told her quickly, "I'm sorry but I think you're mistaken. I don't know who you could mean." The woman turned around and left.

The following day the woman returned to Paulette's home and was told that Paulette wasn't home. Maria asked the construction workers there at the time if they knew what time she would be back. They had no idea. As before, Maria left.

The next day Maria returned again and knocked on the door. Paulette answered. Maria told her again that "The voice in my head says that you are the one who knows Robert and that I am in desperate need to speak with him." This time Paulette ponders for a moment before answering. She remembers that Robert (whom she knows as Bob) is involved with the paranormal. She tells Maria that she will call her sister-in-law Antoinette to see if the Robert she is looking for might be her brother Bob. Paulette learned from Maria that she was walking almost a mile from her home each time precisely to her house because she was guided by a voice that told her Paulette was her connection to Robert.

At that time Robert and Antoinette did not indiscriminately talk about their explorations into the spirit world. Nor did they reveal to many people that while they might know him as Bob, to those in the spirit world he was *Robert*.

Upon hearing of the account from Paulette, Antoinette asked for Maria's phone number. She told Paulette that she would give the information to her brother Bob for his opinion on the matter. He immediately recognized the lead as a possible spiritually related communication and phoned Maria.

Maria told Robert that an inner voice led her to Paulette's house to look for him. Maria told Robert that her life is in shambles. She doesn't know what to do anymore. She was heavily depressed and hated her life. Not explaining about what they did at the time, he asked Maria for her name at birth and birth date. He told her he needed that to find out if there was a way we could help her.

Robert in turn relayed that information to Antoinette so she could pass it on to a Spirit Guide. The next day he visited Antoinette in person so that he could place her in hypnotic trance to make the spiritual connection to Rajah. From their guide at the time named Rajah, he learned that Maria was severely *Attached* and that the *Attachment* is trying to destroy her. It was Maria's guide who sent her to Robert. Rajah adds, "Maria was sexually assaulted fourteen years previously at the age of eighteen. That is also when Maria got *Attached*. This one is bad and we need to remove it as soon as we can."

Robert called Maria with the news and told her not to worry because we can help her. He set up the appointment for her removal the next day. At the time he was working with an intuitive energy medicine practitioner by the name of Lorraine to help me with removals. Lorraine was available and confirmed she would be at the 1 o'clock appointment.

They were all gathered at the appointed hour as planned except Maria. She is late. Finally at 1:45 she shows up with her daughter. Maria informed Robert that she kept getting lost as if there was a force preventing her from getting to the appointment on time. He already knew that it was not unusual for an *Attachment* to exert its influence so that the client could not show up. Therefore this wasn't the first time this happened and it certainly would not be the last.

Robert and his team went ahead and got to work. Robert placed Maria into a light trance state. Per Rajah's guidance, he had Rose Oil on hand. Applying it would help expel the *Attachment*. Antoinette was also placed in trance so that Rajah could be present to guide Lorraine to where the entity was moving throughout Maria's body. This removal took about a half an hour to complete. Rajah tells us that Maria is clear.

It is what happened next that astonished Robert. Once he brought Maria out of trance she blinked a few times and checked to see if she has her glasses on already. When she realized that she wasn't wearing them she exclaims "I can see without my glasses. I can see!" She was just so happy. More than having her vision clear again to the point she could see without her glasses, she felt as if a big heavy weight was now lifted from her shoulders. She expressed feeling free again. Maria spoke for a while longer. She described how her mind was always telling her that she was not good and how her family life was being ruined because of her inadequacy.

As for Robert and his team, this was the first case where they saw a physical ailment go away immediately after removing an *Attachment*. But as with other things, they would see this occur time and time again.

In many *Attachment* cases there had been some previous episode that resulted in mental, emotional, and or physical weaknesses that created the vulnerability to becoming *Attached*. In these cases, such as was the case with Maria, victims are considered to be re-victimized over and over because it is through no fault of her own, but by the *Attachment's* influence, that her life presented additional struggles that may not have occurred to her otherwise.

Sometimes Robert hears back from client's they've helped, but other times not. He's not heard back from Maria in recent years. But experience tells him she will be in touch again if she needs help in the future.

In time, Robert and his team hope to train others to do the same Ghost Remover process. As more people join the team, they too come to realize the true nature of these beings. Even though some of their behavior may appear demon-like, they are not devils or demons but ghosts.

Spirits of the deceased who have, for whatever reason, failed to successfully transition. While Robert and his team can do many other things with the help of the Spirit connections they have established, Robert's strongest passion centers around clearing victims of *Attachments* that have no right affecting, let alone infecting, the living.

Very often it is a family member that seeks help for a loved one who is in distress. In this case a wife confided in her friend, who happened to be the caretaker of a client in an upcoming case, that she was worried about her husband who serves in the military. The caretaker suggested to her that Robert might be able to help. Robert is very interested in helping the military because they put themselves on the line for our country. And, because he is aware that combat situations can also increase their risk to becoming *Attached*.

CASE FILE: Concerned Wife
Robert Major writes:

> Rodney's wife described his occupation as a soldier. She confided that Rodney had become very distant and depressed upon returning from his most recent deployment to Iraq. After explaining to her what we do, she asked that we check to see if he was *Attached*. I did. He was *Attached*. Through our mutual mainstream medical contact, caretaker, we set an appointment with Rodney to do the removal. Upon meeting Rodney I could tell by looking into his eyes that the *Attachments* were quite powerful. Once the *Attachments* are found out, they act nervous. From experience, I recognize their agitation.

Attachments act differently when they encounter us because they realize they are going to be removed. They understand that their presence as they perceive it is coming to an end. They are aware of this because they eavesdrop on the person's thoughts and intentions that they are *Attached* to. *Attachments* have the unique position of having a one-sided intimacy with the person whom they've *Attached*. That person, however, is usually completely unaware, only experiencing the influences of the *Attachments*. Much more than a stalker who observes from afar, *Attachments* become intimately familiar with their host up close and personal.

These misguided entities will be handed over to spirit guides who help them on to their next state in the afterlife. Yet they are often fearful of the transition which could be one reason why they didn't go in the first place. This situation is different than talk therapy which is designed to get the different personalities talking and cooperating. In those cases, if there are *Attachments* present instead of a mental disorder, the *Attachments* do not feel threatened and so they participate. However, when it is time to be removed they behave in ways I now perceive as nervousness patterns.

Now that Rodney was in the office, we were able to determine the number of *Attachments* which was extremely high. There were eighty-one present on Rodney. In multiple *Attachment* cases there are always a few that are the strongest. The others just basically empower those two or three. During the session we learned that Rodney had been *Attached* prior to going to Iraq. There were abusive situations in his youth that created the vulnerability and openings in the Subtle Body that allowed the *Attachments* in at around age nine.

We moved into the removal process. The removals went quite smoothly. Nothing was out of the ordinary in clearing them. Upon completion of the removals I noticed a much more relaxed individual. Rodney was more at peace. He expressed gratitude. He said he felt a lot lighter. Two weeks later I phoned Rodney. He said he felt quite good. Two months later however, Rodney expressed feeling depressed. I checked him again at that time but he was not *Attached* so there was nothing else I or anyone in my team could do because his symptoms were not *Attachment* related.

The following client was referred to Robert by a previous client who now exhibits the ability to perceive ghosts moving in and out of people. In other words, he has demonstrated the ability to recognize the presence of an *Attachment* on others. In Jane's case, he made the observation and referred her to Robert.

CASE FILE: A Nurse Named Jane
Robert writes:

Mike, who had been one of my clients, contacted me to say he was worried about his girlfriend Jane. She was a nurse at a VA hospital and she was having big problems. He felt this *Attachment* was very powerful and was controlling Jane's behavior.

He went on to say the tire on his car was slashed and he thought it might have been Jane's *Attachment* that was responsible. I told him to have her call me with her full name at birth and birth date. Again, this is all that is required for the spirit world to check a person for an *Attachment*. All of your life is filed under that format. With this information we can find out if a person is *Attached*. And, sometimes we can tell just with that information the severity of the *Attachment*. Jane called, provided the information and set an appointment for the following Saturday for a consultation.

It is during the appointment that I am able to get a sense of the *Attachment* and most often, find out how the opening that allowed it to enter originally occurred. I noted that Jane arrived on time. That was an important indicator to me because I have seen instances where the *Attachment* has so much power over the individual that *It* is able to keep the client from meeting with me. That is why I do not attempt to learn anything about the *Attachment* in advance of the appointment. To do so increases the risk of triggering the *Attachment* to act out which could be detrimental to the client.

Jane is a very beautiful young woman in her mid-twenties. I could feel her apprehensiveness when we met. I'm sure she would never have believed in this sort of thing if Mike had not forced the issue. I had Jane take a seat in the office. Note taking during the interview can be distracting and so in some cases, I videotape the session.

We talked about her childhood for a while and then moved on to traumatic times in her life. These are the times I have found when a tear[9] in the energetic field of the Subtle Body can occur resulting in vulnerability to *Attachments*. Jane was pretty open once she knew what I was looking for. She told me she had been raped four years ago. All too often this is how young women get *Attached*. Sexual attacks are a major cause of openings occurring in the Subtle Body.

We talked more about what to expect when we do the removal. I wrote down the address of Antoinette's house to accommodate her scheduling the coming Tuesday. I could tell Jane was just nervous with the whole situation. So, I assured her everything will be just fine. "We always get our ghost." I tell her jokingly to break the ice as I accompany her down the walkway as she left.

I had already gotten information from Antoinette telling me this *Attachment* was a pretty bad one. The next day was Easter and around midday Antoinette phones me saying "You're never going to believe what just happened to me. I went outside the front of the house to sit on the steps to talk on the phone. While I was out there I heard my neighbor's car start-up across the street.

---

[9] Suggested Resource: For images of Subtle Body issues refer to Hands of Light by Barbara Brennan.

Thinking nothing of that I waved only to see the strangest thing happening. There was no one in the car. No driver. It abruptly made a ninety-degree turn and tried to run me down. Luckily for me I was able to get out of the way and the car ended up hitting the house. It didn't do much damage but I was quite shaken." She added, "The police were called and the fire department was here in minutes. The police were suspicious of my story and thought I was covering up for my neighbor. I told them that was not the case. I had no reason to lie. The police were baffled. I could see that. One officer spoke up and said 'Maybe it was a ghost.' I wondered about that."

"Two days later we would find out the truth." Antoinette continues. "That policeman didn't know how right he was. It was a ghost that had taken control of the vehicle which was parked, locked and empty at the time it started up and attempted to take me out."

Robert recounts what happened next. "We met at the house that following Tuesday for Jane's removal. I showed up early so I can cover any variables that might occur. I placed Antoinette into hypnotic trance so that she could connect to the Spirit world. Once she was in trance she moved aside in the normal way for whichever spirit guide that is to come in. Rajah was there that day and spoke first. She told us that it was the ghost who caused all the commotion on Sunday and that the ghost was trying to scare Antoinette from doing the removal. Had Antoinette not made it up the front porch steps and out of the way of the oncoming vehicle that was coming upon her in the front yard, the situation could have been a lot worse. Antoinette has had items flying about her house, been choked by ghosts, and *Attached* herself more than once so she does not scare easily. But the event with the vehicle that day shook her up."

Sometimes things are needed for the removal. Rajah told us rose petals would be necessary for this removal. Team member Marcos headed down the street to find a rose. I had the client lie on a basic massage table for removals. That way the Ghost Remover can maneuver around the person if needed. These ghostly energies can be very tricky and we cannot slip up once we are in the removal process. If *It* escapes *It* can jump, what is referred to as 'body-hop' to another persona and *Attach* again if we're not careful.

Rajah tells us that the opening is primarily around the navel area with a slight opening around the left thigh. That is where I will extract from. About the time Jane arrives, Marcos returns with a rose. Jane sat on the massage table. I immediately put Jane into a light trance and then had her lie back on the table. As Rajah instructed, I placed the rose petals around her navel and thigh. Once everyone was in position I began the removal. As I started pulling the entity from the navel region I hear Jane start to yell, "It's burning! It's burning!"

The entity wasn't leaving without a fight. The *Attachment* was female. *She* was trying to move all round the body to avoid being removed. But we were able to capture her. With eyes closed, Marcos can sense the Ghost move throughout Jane's body. He tracked it. I captured it and handed it over to Marcos who in turn handed it over to the Spirit Guide who was waiting to receive it.

Rajah had already told me that this ghost was a young woman named Esther. Esther was a young woman of African descent who committed suicide in 1976 at the age of twenty-three. She was from a broken home and had become a prostitute. Rajah told us that Esther would most likely be given another chance after being re-educated in the spirit world. We were previously told that we are all considered 'children' until we reach twenty-four years of age. Since Esther was so young at the time she took her own life she would be able to keep her soul and someday return to live another earthly existence. Spirit Guides have told me that this is not always the case. There are times a spirit will have to surrender its soul and will no longer exist. From our experience, that is sometimes the case but only under certain circumstances. But when they are, I am told that the soul is sent back to a pool of 'energy'. A kind of wellspring from which another personality can come forth and develop.

Like most removals, Jane's took no more than thirty minutes. We did a final check after the clearing to make sure there are no remnants and do not end the session until we get the 'all-clear' signal from the Spirit Guide. Afterwards, I let Jane remain lying on the massage table for a few minutes to rest. At the time of this removal we did not have our aura sealer, Daniel. He wasn't to come to us for another year.

Before ending the session, I told Jane she needed to be very careful because she still had the openings in her aura. She told me that she was heading to New Orleans the following week. I told her that she needed to be careful about drinking and concentrate on closing those openings that Rajah identified. Not surprisingly, upon Jane's return from New Orleans we checked her and found she had been *Attached* again. That gets frustrating for us. Luckily this next *Attachment* was nothing like Esther but *It* could have been. I scheduled and performed another removal the following week. All went fine. After Daniel joined our team, we could seal the openings in the Subtle Body. I had Jane come back for a session with Daniel so that he could close up the openings that existed in her aura. Daniel sealed the openings. During my follow-up with Jane weeks later she told me that she has her life back to herself again and thanked us for that.

Understandably, when people hear about the Ghost Removers and what they do there can be skepticism. However, people turn to them when conventional means have not provided relief. A man named Aaron had come upon the Ghost Removers and decided to get checked for the presence of an *Attachment* because nothing he'd tried up to that point could alleviate the chronic pain he had in his knee. It turned out that in this case the *Attachment* itself was causing the pain. Once Aaron was cleared of the *Attachment* he was relieved of the pain. This is a great example that helps clarify an important point. The Ghost Removers don't cure anything. What problems a person had before the clearing remain. What is gone is any issue the *Attachment* brought in with it. In Aaron's case, it was the pain in his knee. From then on Aaron followed the Ghost Removers via their website. The following case was referred to Robert by Aaron.

CASE FILE: Referrals from Aaron

Like other clients, as a result of his *Attachment* removal, Aaron could sense *Attachments* on others. That is what led him to implore an entire family (Jane, her husband George, daughter Sue, son Larry and Jane's mother Agnes) to seek out the help of the Ghost Removers. However, Aaron had trouble explaining what it is that Robert and his team actually did. As a result, all he could do was encourage them to give it a try.

Jane writes about her experience:

> I took my family to see Robert and Antoinette in May. The experience was so profound I wanted to share our family's story with them. As a result of the *Attachment* removal, I feel they have helped me and my family so much. Robert and Antoinette are angels themselves.
>
> The main reason I brought my daughter, Sue to the appointment was because she'd been having health issues for two years. She had two surgeries for a tumor in her head. But even after the surgeries, she had trouble with sleep, focusing, and expressed feeling crazy. Every time we've gone to the doctor

to try to figure out why all they could tell me is that she's a mystery. During the appointment with Robert, we found out that my daughter was *Attached* by two ghosts. They were interfering with Sue's sleep, concentration, and focus. They caused her anxiety. Since the removal, she is so much better and expresses feeling better. The changes I see regarding those issues are amazing to me. I wish I would have known about Robert and Antoinette years ago. I cannot help but feel that my daughter's life would have been easier without the influence of the *Attachments*. Sue is still working on her sleep issues but reports everything else is better.

As for myself, I found out during the same appointment that I was *Attached* by two ghosts. In my case, I'd been plagued by high blood pressure for the last eight months which registered 198/94. At times, I felt like I was having a heart attack. This occurred quite often. There were times when I found myself in a state of being very sad. During these times I would worry and cry. Not just a little, but a lot. The worry would escalate and intensify until I felt like I was making myself crazy. After having the *Attachments* removed, I felt better, even that day. So I checked my blood pressure a few hours after the removal. It was 123/76. I feel so much better!

My son Larry was at the appointment too. His issue stemmed from chronic shoulder pain. After he was cleared of the *Attachment,* his shoulder hasn't hurt him since. As for my husband George, we learned, was *Attached* by seven! After getting them removed,

I find things are so much better. While he didn't notice a lot of difference, my kids and I see a huge difference. We find George easier to talk to.

Here's the weird thing about George's removal. When Antoinette removed one of the *Attachments* the room smelled really bad. I immediately recalled how George's shirts and bath towel would have the same sour bad smell. Two days after the removal, I realized that the smell was no longer on him or in the house. It was completely gone.

The last removal was on my mom, Agnes who is 85 years old. She has Alzheimer's and it's been a terrible thing to have anyway as anyone affected by that disease will tell you. I'm not saying here that the Ghost Removers can cure Alzheimer's, but their work has made our life with mom easier in a few respects. My mom was *Attached* by seven and since they were removed I find that I'm now just dealing with the Alzheimer's. It is only by their absence that I realize I was dealing with the *Attachments* too. Alzheimer's related symptoms are still a very hard thing to deal with in regards to the short-term memory problems. But since the clearing, I find she's a lot nicer.

With the benefit of hindsight, I now understand that it was the *Attachments* that caused my mom to appear weird to me at times when she would totally change in front of me. She would hunch over, her eyes would change, her face would become very wrinkled. Her behavior changed during these episodes too. Sometimes she would be very suspicious. Or she would fight with me and get in my face. Other times, she could be quite amusing.

Agnes complained about a pain she had in the top of her head. It plagued her 24/7. Since the removal, that pain in her head is gone which is amazing to me. And, this last shift was unique. In the past, when we would go out shopping, she would steal. We had to go to court one time for that. Just the other day, after a shopping trip, she told me, "You know, when I'm in the store and I'm shopping I don't hear that voice anymore that told me to 'Take It. Take It. You want to take it!'" Not only is my family feeling better overall, but everyone in our family is so much closer. As a result, the whole house has a different feel to it. It's a lot lighter. We have never been happier as a family. Thanks again Robert and Antoinette.

Sincerely,
Jane

As we've seen in these cases, people struggle with many different issues. *Attachments* jump in where they can and create problems layered on top of what people are already challenged with. It is the Ghost Remover's view that we should all have the opportunity to face our own problems without the extra burden the *Attachments* inflict. Their influence may not even be realized as in the case of Jane's family, until they are gone. Understanding the nature of the problem and why it is so prevalent will go a long way to alleviating it.

CHAPTER 8:
THE NATURE OF
SEVERE
ATTACHMENTS

A severe *Attachment* is the term Robert Major uses to describe a ghost who's activity has escalated to the point where it seeks to use a living person in a parasitic relationship to satisfy its own needs. In that and other ways, *Attachments* are a form of *parasitism*. Parasitism is defined as a non-mutual symbiotic relationship where the parasite benefits at the expense of the host. Unlike predators, parasites do not kill their host, and will often live in or on their host for an extended period of time. Classic examples of parasitism include tapeworms and fleas.

Parasites are known for reducing a host's biological fitness by general or specialized pathology. Parasites increase their own fitness by exploiting hosts for resources. Parasitic qualities apply to *Attachments*. In the case of ghosts that *Attach*, they can gain strength, even thrive, while the host is receding. An example of a ghost who fueled itself off of pain energy can be found in the following Ghost Remover case file.

CASE FILE: Frank the Architect

This author recalls:

> A young man named Frank, in his twenties at the time, had an *Attachment* removed by the team. During the removal process Antoinette learned from Rajah the *Attachment* had been on him since around age 4. It was at that age that an event occurred that created the original vulnerability to being *Attached* and that *It* fed off of pain energy. She revealed this information to Frank who said that there had been a 'situation' around that time. He revealed that he remembers clearly that his father had brutally beat him when he was only four years old. With the benefit of hindsight Frank now realized that event was a turning point in his life. He went on to say that from that point forward he was accident prone. Starting with snow skiing accidents in his youth, to auto accidents in his teenage years and a skydiving accident in his early twenties, at one point or another, he had ended up breaking nearly every bone in his body. As a result, Frank was now in constant pain.
>
> After the removal, Frank was sensitive to perceiving *Attachments* on others. He assisted on at least one removal a few weeks after his own clearing. This author was there and lent a hand. Suddenly I felt the energy grow extremely cold so I mentioned it. Frank said he found the *Attachment* reluctant to go and so he infused it with cold energy to freeze it so we could then remove it in its entirety. It worked.
>
> Frank checks in with Robert occasionally and

reports that even now, nearly a decade after being cleared of his *Attachment* he has not had any accidents.

The Ghost Remover team know what the *Attachments* are doing and how they do it because they too are able to traverse these realms safely. The difference between spirits of the dead and the Ghost Remover team members is intention. Ghosts seek to benefit themselves (even at the expense of another) and spirit guides desire to help others. These pure intentions are essential to the Ghost Remover team's success.

In some instances, a powerful *Attachment* can inflict a heavy toll on a person's life.

CASE FILE: "Mike's Not Here"
Robert Major writes:

> Awhile back I was called on by Dave to see what was going on with a friend named Mike. Dave went on to say that Mike, an engineer for a big corporation, had taken to "partying heavily". He recently cleared out his bank account and given all of the money away. He added that he moved all of his furnishings in the house onto the lawn and put a "Free" sign up for everything. He gave his car to a neighbor down the street and started preaching the word of God. The police picked him up mid-day barefoot in shorts and t-shirt clutching a Bible and rambling in the streets in traffic incoherently. Mike was taken to county mental health. He spent three days there before being released.

A few days passed and Mike was home again. I went by his house ... I saw Mike in the distance and when he turned around I noticed right away it wasn't him present. He came up to me and I put out my hand to shake his saying "Hi Mike." Right away I heard this strange voice answering back "Mike's not here. I'm in control now. I never liked that loud mouth anyway. You had better leave." There was nothing for me to do at that moment and so I left.

Dave had informed me that Mike's parents were apprised of the issues and decided to make the trip from Maryland to San Diego to investigate and support their son. Through Dave I learned that Mike's parents were very religious. Often, people have trouble hearing about this type of work because they feel it conflicts with their religious beliefs. In order to reassure them, I wrote a five page letter to explain what we do and let them know I felt I could help Mike. But, I needed to put it more in a religious context so they could digest the information. I incorporated information from the Bible that I thought could offer them insight into what was about to occur in the session.

When I heard they were in town, I asked to meet with them a few days before the removal. They were somewhat apprehensive but they had very few options. Therefore they were willing to try anything and were willing to let us proceed. However, they chose not to attend the removal session.

Lorraine, who is also an energy healer, did this

removal. Lorraine was the best we had at the time. It was a tough removal. This was the first time I was able to speak with one of the entities. The Spirit Guide Rajah spoke through Antoinette and asked me, "Would you like to converse with this entity?" I said "Yes."

It spoke through Antoinette. The first words were, "Who the Fuck do you think you are?" I was somewhat startled, but I responded quickly, "I'm the guy who's going to get you out of here."

Some entities have more vitality and exhibit a stronger sense of consciousness than others. These appear more self aware and are better able to communicate. Those that do can oftentimes recall their names and personal history from when they were living, more so than the weaker ones.

When the entity spoke again he told us that his name was Carl. We were to find out that he, and the other two entities that were controlling Mike had lived in the 1930's and 1940's. They are best described as alcoholic hobos. Each had died from cirrhosis of the liver. Carl was the leader and the other two were empowering him with their energy.

Just as a person can have more than one spirit guide, they can likewise be *Attached* by more than one ghost. Sometimes they *Attach* to a human host at the same moment in time. In other cases, one *Attaches* first. Then others are attracted to either the host or the *Attachment*. They can easily find the way to *Attach* using the same entry point as the previous entity. Multiple *Attachments* are not uncommon.

As Rajah instructed, there were two "containers" in the room that day. Pat and Dave were part of the team to contain the entities so that they could not escape during the removal process.

The first two *Attachments* were easy for Lorraine to remove. But the third, who had been hiding, was difficult to remove. It took Lorraine probably ten minutes to corral that entity and remove it. Rajah did the final check to make sure that we had gotten all of the *Attachment's* energies that were present.

Mike was 100% immediately back to the person I knew after the *Attachment* removal. As soon as I looked into Mike's eyes I could see only his presence. That was when I was sure he was completely "back". In the weeks that followed, Mike was evasive in his recognition of what had happened during the Ghost Remover process. He wanted to equate it to devils and demons in more of a religious context. And, he still does that to this day. Mike's parents were happy their son was back but the whole process was too overwhelming for their religious point of view. In retrospect, the seemingly strange world of ghosts and *Attachments* was perceived as possibly being antithetical to their most deeply held religious convictions. I have not heard from them since.

Often it is not known what the original traumas are that lead people like Mike to abuse substances that ultimately lead them to getting *Attached*. However,

Robert and his team see that type of scenario all the time.

Since Mike's removal he has exhibited the ability to see ghosts moving in and out of people. Based on client feedback, it is often the case that a cleared person can perceive *Attachments*. Several Ghost Remover team members were at one time, cleared of *Attachments* by our team. A year after Mike's removal he phoned in a referral to a friend he'd identified as being *Attached*.

Mike's case was not unique in that many people experiment with substance abuse as a means of escaping their reality. As they become 'intoxicated', their own spirit departs their body which has become too toxic for it to inhabit. In doing so, they create an opening in their Subtle Body which serves as a protective energetic field. An intruder of like energy to the toxic substance may seize the opportunity to *Attach*. An earlier physical, mental, or emotional trauma which previously affected Subtle Body anatomy and appears on that level was likely the impetus for substance abusing in the first place. It is that vulnerability in the Subtle Body that is referred to when speaking about weakness that leads to vulnerability to becoming *Attached*.

In cases where one actually passes out, when they return to their body, it is often still in the stages of clearing out the toxins. So, the addition of an *Attachment* often goes unnoticed. In some cases, the *Attachment* adjusts its influence to mimic symptoms already present to avoid being detected. Relapsing into substance abuse time and time again increases the probability of becoming *Attached* by one or multiple *Attachments* exponentially. Multiple

Attachments occur because the current *Attachment(s)* are refueled and so drive the addictive behavior which weakens the host and makes it easier for more *Attachments* to enter. The ability of the *Attachment(s)* to affect or infect the host increases with each re-use.

Susceptibility to *Attachment(s)* can occur from physical, mental, and/or emotional trauma. In these cases, the person is walking around with an existing vulnerability, and it is only a matter of time before they up in a situation which can be exploited by an *Attachment.*

CASE FILE: A Visit to the Doctor

A few years ago Sheila incurred a traumatic brain injury. Her cognitive deficits and brain damage were well documented in her medical file. Because certain cognitive stimulus was shown to cause her brain to go into seizure she made sure each new doctor she was sent to was aware of this vulnerability to avoid accidentally triggering it. Here's her account of what happened when she was sent to a new doctor for assessment.

> The doctor looked at me from across his desk. His mouth did not move, yet I clearly heard the words, "I'm going to break you." At first, I thought this was some kind of a joke. I quickly glanced around his office to see if I was on a hidden camera show or something trippy like that. I immediately realized however, that this was no joke. To my shock and horror this doctor immediately replicated the same stimulus described in my medical report that confirmed would result in seizure. It did.
>
> In the weeks that followed basic activities of daily

living became increasingly more challenging. It became difficult to get through the day at all. At times, I'd briefly blackout. The need for sleep both day and night increased but I experienced a profound inability to feel rested. Every night I was haunted by the experience of reliving the incident in the doctor's office. From lack of restful sleep and mental duress, I was going downhill fast.

At times I was so weak I often wondered if it was easier to give up and die. Other times, I pictured myself leaving the house and going homeless. I saw images of myself finding a place outside where I could sleep on the ground outdoors. Forever! In the past, I would never have allowed such thoughts into my head. However, I was so weary, escape by any means seemed to beckon me from an unknown source.

About six weeks into it, I had awoken about 2 am to go to the bathroom. I went down on the cold hard tiled living room floor but was not blacked out. Instead, I'd lost all motor control. I could not move nor speak. At 8am my roommate found me and drove me to Urgent Care. Within minutes of arriving they had teams of people all around me. My blood pressure reading was over 250. I was incapacitated as if paralyzed, yet I was aware of a flurry of staff activity all around me. I was sent by ambulance to the E.R. Nothing could be diagnosed. I had regained my ability to speak and move. My blood pressure returned to normal and so I was discharged.

The turning point occurred when I was confirmed as having an *Attachment* and then cleared of it by Robert Major and Ghost Remover Marcos.

Without knowing anything about my situation, during the session Marcos told me, "These *Attachments* were on the doctor. They had been seeking a suitable host and saw the doctor as a conduit for them to find just the right victim with the vulnerability and body that they wanted. When you came in, they targeted you. *They* took over and possessed the doctor. *They* did that to you that day. *They* wanted to take you out."

When I shared my experience with Marcos while I was at the E.R. and the recent spike in blood pressure Marcos said that it was just one of the ways the *Attachments* were using to get *me* to leave. They wanted *my* body. And, they wanted to live homeless, out on the streets.

That news sent chills down the back of my neck as I recalled the feelings I'd been having of wanting to escape into the anonymity of living homeless on the streets. In the recent weeks that had become an increasingly secret desire I'd shared with no one.

During the removal, when it came time to go, they did not want to be removed, but Ghost Remover Marcos was steadfast in clearing them from me. Marcos described the dark nature of the *Attachment* to me as a kind of dark caricatures, bat like, flying out of my head. In less than twenty minutes, they were gone. I felt myself, my own spirit, pouring back into body. *They* were no longer there. I knew that. The shift was immediate and profound.

At the completion of the removal process with Marcos and Robert I noticed immediately that I now had energy flowing into my hands and feet. As it did, I got my mobility back. Marcos commented, "Of course. The human energy field (aka Subtle Body) acts as an immune system. In my case, what the human energy field did in response to these severe *Attachments,* was to contain the *Attachments* where they were in my brain. This meant that I had no energy in my limbs which is why I was losing motor control and experiencing lapses in consciousness. The sensation is similar getting out of a chair and finding one's leg asleep. While numb, it is nearly impossible to walk normally. Once the circulation returns, so does the movement.

The energy field immune response that I experienced is exemplified in the case of needing to sleep after ingesting a huge Thanksgiving dinner. All energy is diverted to digestion which results in a 'food coma'. In my case however, all energy was diverted to containment of the invading *Attachments* in my brain and so I was experiencing a similar coma reaction but more on the scale of my limbs being asleep in the rest of my body.

Ever since the removal, I no longer heard the doctor's voice in my head and was no longer haunted by the episode.

Not everyone who has had a concussion will get *Attached,*

but one client did. Like others, this client now understands from first-hand experience that previous traumas makes her vulnerable to *Attachments*. Therefore, she checks in with the Ghost Removers whenever she feels 'not herself'. On two subsequent occasions, she had become re-*Attached* and the Ghost Removers cleared her of these as well.

Attachment cases are often complicated. Sometimes people seek out the Ghost Removers because they or a loved one have a problem that has been irresolvable by conventional means. Robert and his team offer their help. Sometimes it is accepted. Other times it is refused. As a result, sometimes the Ghost Remover team is not able to help.

CASE FILE: Multiple *Attachments*
Robert Major writes:

> The parents of a young man contacted me out of desperation. Their son, in his twenties, had fathered several children by different women in several states around the United States. He had restraining orders against him. He has had several bouts with the law and criminal justice system. Also, he has been unable to get or keep a steady job. We discovered that he had the most *Attachments* on one person we had ever seen up to that point in time (about 2012): thirty-six.

> I was caught off guard at our meeting because I was preoccupied when he reached out his hand. Without thinking, I reached out and shook it. I felt one of the *Attachments* jump on to me. I got cleared of it right away. Unfortunately, the young man was not open to receiving our assistance to clear him.

Whether it was actually the young man himself who refused a clearing or one of the *Attachments* stepping in to refuse it we cannot say for sure because we did not check that. We cannot proceed without the consent of the person presenting in the body. I'm sorry to say he remains *Attached* to this day.

In the case of the young man who has the most *Attachments* but will not authorize a removal, Robert can only stand by hoping for an opportunity to arise in which he can help him sometime in the future. As time goes by Robert hears second-hand accounts of this man's relationship problems escalating. He is reported to have fathered more children with different women and continues to commit crimes that land him in the hands of the authorities.

Like an innocent fugitive, a severely *Attached* person is driven to seek out new relationships, employment and places to live on a regular basis to avoid having to explain their issues or account for past misdeeds while the *Attachment* was 'In'. Their transient behavior allows the *Attachment* to go undetected. But on the other hand, they cannot maintain an ordinary social life. Therefore, it is difficult for the person to advance in their work because the *Attachment* eventually emerges in each new situation, making it necessary for him to leave positions, even those with promise. As a result, the person is forced to restart over and over at the worst and lowest paying jobs which eventually leaves the person with a lack of self confidence, a feeling of hopelessness and a sense that the world is against him. If he has children, even if he loves them, he is unable to be a reliable parent to any degree. The *Attachments* find no passion nor compassion for a family not of their

126

own making. He can find no way out of the problems which continue to mount with each passing day.

The human host is driven remain in the comfort of their own community and family. The *Attachment*, on the other hand, desires the anonymity inherent in a difficult and complicated transitory lifestyle. The *Attachments* seeks dysfunctional associations so that they can get 'Out' unnoticed with people and in places unfamiliar to the host.

Responsibility, materialism and wealth in the way we normally think of them do not matter to an *Attachment* unless of course, they are viewed as a means to an ends for their sole benefit. That means they are unconcerned with what is considered normal life issues such as a healthy concern for self and others, education, making a living and so forth *because they are not of this three-dimensional world.* Nor are they constrained by time and space in the way someone born into this world is. For these reasons, they are self-centered, self-serving, and uncompassionate spirits who are vying to gain control of the physical body to the point that eventually, they, *and only they,* are the only one 'In' on a permanent basis. Until such time, they seek every opportunity to lead what fragment of a life they can.

Ghosts may linger around certain areas. There are different reasons for this. They may have died there, as in a battle or famine or from disease, or they may be drawn to a location by the presence of other ghosts. They may not understand their predicament nor realize that help is available.

In other situations, very often the people ghosts victimize and are seeking help don't understand what is happening, or simply have run out of options. The Ghost Removers even get calls from those in the medical community who discretely refer clients to them and request that they and their clients remain anonymous. In one such instance, the bizarre behavior of a patient was a telltale sign to a caretaker familiar with Robert's work that there could be an *Attachment* present. She therefore contacted Robert in regards to someone she felt desperately needed his help.

CASE FILE: Self-Cannibalism
Robert Major writes:

> A caretaker for a young woman came to us concerned about the lady she cared for who was often physically restrained because she would bite and eat her own flesh, especially on her arms. The caretaker reported that in some places on her forearms she chewed to the bone. The damage she did to herself was horrible. When we cleared this woman of her *Attachment*, we discovered that it was the ghosting spirit of a cannibal along with six other spirits of people he had cannibalized when he was alive. The image we got of the cannibal as he left revealed that he prized his teeth which he had filed down to points during that lifetime. Since being cleared of this *Attachment* and the one's he brought in with him, the young woman ceased cannibalizing herself.
>
> After so many years of experience, it has become apparent that the uncharacteristic behavior exhibited by the client is likely a signpost as to the personality of the *Attachment(s)*. In the case of this young woman, she was *Attached* by both the cannibal *and* six of its victims. Since she acted out

upon herself, she had exhibited both the perpetrator and victim patterns. Had the <u>victims</u> not been *Attached,* it is doubtful she would have cannibalized and mutilated <u>herself.</u>

In multiple follow-ups with the caretaker in the weeks, months and now years since the *Attachment* removal, the woman has been symptom free.

In this case, the strange nature of the behavior offered insight into the nature of the *Attachment's* personality. The bizarre type of behavior exhibited by the self-cannibalizer in the not too distant past might have been categorized under the antiquated medical term known as *hysteria.* A diagnosis of *hysteria* was assigned to a patient who's symptoms or signs of illness were generally believed to be the result of unconscious emotional or psychological forces within the patient. If there was a period where there was loss of awareness of one's identity during a *hysterical* episode they might have been diagnosed as having *hysterical dissociation.* Currently, there is no western medical term for *Attachment* but there should be.

CHAPTER 9:
ATTACHMENT SCENARIOS:
CASES OF A DIFFERENT KIND

It is helpful to understand that anyone can become *Attached*. The following Ghost Remover case files are accounts of how ordinary people became vulnerable and ended up becoming *Attached* as well as highlighting other skills of Ghost Remover team members.

CASE FILE: Robb the Artist Part I – Animal Communication
Written by Robb, a middle aged man, who refers to Robert Major as Bob in his account that follows. The first segment involves animal communication and the second part is about his *Attachment* case. Combined, they offer a unique perspective into other talents.

> I first met Bob Major at my favorite place in San Diego, Cass Street Bar and Grill in Pacific Beach. I immediately got along with Bob as he and I shared a love for animals, people and for helping others. After I had spent many hours talking with Bob over pool games, burgers and chicken salads he offered me his assistance with my animals. At the

time, I had over 45 animals, which I kept as educational animal ambassadors for the art and science classes I teach throughout San Diego. Bob explained to me that he and his sister Antoinette could do animal communication along with help of a couple of their 'gifted' friends.

At first, I had my doubts but wanted to keep an open mind. I immediately wanted to find out more about my two collies and St. Bernard, the most cherished of my menagerie. Bob asked me to write down as many questions that I wanted information about, really anything I wanted to know. A week later, I drove to Bob's sister's house with Miles and Belle, my standard collies and Bigs the St. Bernard, and a multitude of questions in hand.

Once we began the session I could instantly feel the dog's presence in the room (they were just outside in my car, as they only need to be within a 100 yards for the communication to work). I was amazed at some of the answers as they were completely non-coincidental. Bob has never been to my current house and although we are friends, he did not know the exact details of my dogs' lives. I was able to question my dogs at length and discovered that Bigs wanted to know why I don't get him big bones anymore which I had actually stopped buying because they were too expensive. Also, he said there is a guy who always comes over and yells at them and I found out later there was a neighbor who did just that. Many more questions and answers I found were things that actually fit what I knew was true about my dogs.

The animal communication was lengthy. In summary Rob continues: Bob, or really anyone other than those who currently live with me did not previously know these factors. After this session, I brought more of my animals and receive more amazing responses from them. My giant monitor lizard asked me for more bloody meat as I had previously been feeding him fresh mackerel. He also threatened to make turtle soup out of his upstairs neighbor (my baby African tortoise who lived in the tank above him in the garage). My frogs asked for more fruit flies and I had been feeding them crickets instead for quite a while. My big tortoise Art explained how he had lost part of his shell by being stuck under something when he got out, (he was caught under a car). These experiences and many others have caused me to suspend my disbelief and gain full respect for the abilities of Bob, Antoinette and their group.

CASE FILE: Robb the Artist Part II – *Attachment*
Robb the Artist writes:

> Years later, I was in need of Bob's help. It was NFL playoff weekend, and things hadn't been right for me for quite some time. I had heard stories of Bob doing ghost removals from people who had ghosts *"Attach"* themselves to them, usually only to cause harm to their lives. Although I was again a bit skeptical of this, I had to keep an open mind. I mentioned to Bob that I had been angry, drinking a LOT of hard alcohol, drinking and driving, getting into fights with people, all very uncharacteristic of me and I had also a lot of bad things happening like things getting stolen, animals dying and complete strangers getting very angry and even

violent with me. Bob asked for my complete name and date of birth, which he gave to his sister, Antoinette to do a reading on (to assess whether or not I was *Attached*). The next Monday, within 24 hours he told me that I had been *Attached* while in San Francisco, the second week of November, when I was drinking in the airport bar. Once again, I do not see or talk to Bob all the time, we are friends but only talk every couple weeks and he does not know the complete details of my life. That weekend I missed my flight to Seattle and had a layover in San Fran, was drinking and depressed over the news of my mother's recent stroke. Even stranger he told me it (the *Attachment*) was an Italian Mafia hit man who had been killed in the 70's by the Chinese mafia at 36 (my current age) and that he wanted to come to San Diego and saw an opening through an injured and intoxicated soul.

Now this is all a little hard to believe for me, or anyone for that matter, but I had to do something to get my life back from its downward spiral and a ghost removal/cleansing session with Bob seemed in good order. Bob had also warned me about one other thing: This ghost hated my animals and wanted to harm them. I made an appointment for Thursday, 3 days later, and anxiously waited. The next day my beloved St. Bernard, Bigs had to be rushed into surgery for stomach bloat and splenectomy. Unfortunately, he did not live through the surgery. The day after that my Hedgehog, Tatertot was dead in his cage. I had only 3 hours until my appointment and things were getting worse. I felt sick and had a terrible headache. While walking my collies Miles and Belle, Miles suddenly began to limp. I thought "Crap! What next??!!" I rushed him home and checked his leg to find no serious injury. Concerned yet running late for my appointment I quickly grabbed some things and rushed to Bob's office.

I arrived to find Bob with two of his associates, one of them Marcos who I had worked with before and to me one of the most gifted of the group. Bob acts as the mediator and communicates through Marcos who speaks to the other side. Through communication I found that this "*Attachment*" had in fact caused many of the ill effects in my recent life. Believe what you will but things had been anything but normal in the past few months and Bob had even warned me about what it wanted to do to my animals. The ghost denied responsibility for what happened to Bigs and I would like to believe this, although his death was a freak occurrence that nobody can find an accurate reason for. During the end of my session, they asked if I had any other questions. I wanted to know what was wrong with my collie Miles and if Bigs was O.K. Bigs was there in spirit and wanted me to know that Miles had a broken toenail on his back left foot and that it was hurting him. He also wanted me to know that he knew he was lucky to have me as an owner and that he would be back again, as a bigger dog, and that I would be his owner.

I returned home feeling light and relaxed. I looked at myself in the mirror and it seemed that my expression had changed from an angry scowl that I had been sporting to a calm and tranquil gaze. I immediately checked my collie Miles' toenail and got goose bumps when I saw exactly what Marcos told me Bigs had said. Miles' back left foot had a broken nail, all the way up to the quick.

These experiences have left me with proof beyond doubt that Bob Major and his associates have an amazing gift that few possess. Believe what you will, and decide for yourself whether it is true or not, I know that it is and that is all the proof I need.

There are many instances where someone just happened to be at the wrong place at the wrong time and got *Attached* as Robb did in the airport. Sometimes there are situations where entire families are *Attached* and it turns out to stem from a location that is haunted as in the following account.

CASE FILE: A Family Affair
Robert Major's contribution along with those of others involved in the case are interwoven to offer a broader perspective on the same situation.

"This case developed over a five year period.", recalls Robert. "It began when a man named Charles came to me wanting to communicate with his grandson Taylor. Taylor had died in a automobile accident." Details of that story relate to another subject matter. Details of that chronicle will be revealed in an upcoming chapter.

In time, Robert learned after checking on them that

both of Charles's daughters, one son-in-law and three grandchildren, were all *Attached*. This account starts with Charles's granddaughter. Brittany had been known by their family as a sweet girl while growing up, however, at 15 years of age, she changed. Now age 18, she had been acting out for three years. She was fighting with her mom all the time. There did not seem to be a clear incident that could account for the changes the family was witnessing in her.

Charles had been introduced to Robert years earlier and had become familiar with his work. This led to Robert's and Antoinette's guest appearance on his radio show to communicate with audience member's pets that they brought into the studio. Now Charles contacted Robert regarding his concerns about his granddaughter.

After checking Brittany for the presence of an *Attachment*, Robert learned from the Spirit Guide that she was seriously *Attached*. In most cases, the Spirit Guide does not expand on the qualities of the *Attachments*, but in this case he did. The ghost had been on her for a number of years and it was causing her behavior to get increasing negative.

Brittany's family had been perplexed by the confrontational behavior she exhibited that was so out of character for her in the past. In time, they became very concerned.

An appointment was made with Brittany and the Ghost Removers were able to do a successful removal. It appeared that that would be the end of it. However, the situation turned out to be more complex. After Brittany's session she went home. When Brittany went into her room strange things started happening. They continued into the night. Her mom phoned the next morning and left this voicemail.

June 3rd: Heather's Voice Mail to Robert

"Hi Bob, This is Heather, Brittany's mom. I wanted to talk to you. Some strange things happened here at the house in the middle of the night. One of our doors was shaking violently. And then all of a sudden all of my daughter's old dolls from when she was little, flew out of a big closet where I had stored them which was closed, and crashed to the floor. Nothing else moved."

"Also, when Brittany woke up this morning, she had two scratches on her face and two on her neck. This is all very weird to me and I don't know what to tell her."

"Since the removal, she's doing really well. She feels great. But she is concerned now because she thinks there are others coming after her. I'm not so sure. Maybe it's related to a scary movie we watched last night. But at the same time I don't have any explanation so I thought I would touch base with you for your thoughts about what is going on here. Please call me."

Robert and several of the team members went out to their house to investigate. Brittany said she'd heard her name being called but when she'd look to see, no one was there. The house, which has one story with a basement, is in a Southeastern California community situated on a large corner lot. Most of the paranormal activity, they say, is happening in the basement. The basement was sectioned off from the main house. The entry was behind a series of shed type doors. Behind the doors was just a dirt floor because there was no foundation to the home. Upon entering, team members noticed a smell that, from previous experience, had become associated with the presence of ghosts. Robert learned that there were many other ghosts in the house. Some were waiting to *Attach* to Brittany. These ghosts were now telling the Ghost Removers that they were really upset that they had cleared her of a ghost. The team went about clearing the house and property of ghosts. But, the story didn't end there either.

During another unrelated session, Rajah, the spirit guide, came in to tell them that Brittany had skills that could add to the team. Robert extended an offer to Brittany to intern with them. She eagerly agreed and began to work as an understudy to seasoned Ghost Removers.

A year went by. Heather, her husband Ray, and their daughter Brittany moved to Texas. Heather's sister Sharon was working with realtors to show Heather's house. But real estate agents who had come to preview the house during the realtor open house said they'd never show the place to client's because of a foul smell. That was not good news to

Sharon who wanted the house to sell quickly. Sharon decided to call Robert about the problem to see if the stench was ghost related.

Upon arriving, Robert and his team found that the area was full of ghosts again. But, they were not the same ghosts as before. These spirits had moved in after the others had gone. Robert, Marcos and Antoinette cleared the area. Apparently there were lots of deaths and killings in that area during the 1800's. Since Heather and Ray moved to Texas, seven or eight ghosts had moved in. They invited others. When the team arrived, there were almost two hundred ghosts who had gathered there. They were glad the home was vacant of living human residents so that they could have the place to themselves. "Sometimes living humans bother us as much as we bother them.", said one ghost. Another ghost threatened one of the team saying, "I'll jump on and *Attach* to YOU!" "I'll go home with YOU!" The Ghost Remover team cleared that one first. By the end of two hours, the area was clear. All the ghosts were moved on. And, there was no longer any smell in the house.

Sharon phoned the realtors and encouraged them to return. She had a rough time convincing them that the issue was resolved. Skeptical, they reluctantly came back to the house. When they did, they reacted in amazement as they found the bad smell was indeed, completely gone after all. They could not account for the drastic change. Sharon did not volunteer the real explanation as to why it had changed because it didn't seem like the kind of thing they would be receptive to hearing.

East San Diego County has its share of ghosts. And so it was not a surprise when Robert learned that, like Heather's home, Sharon's place needed to be cleared as well. The Ghost Remover team was in the process of clearing Sharon's home when things took yet another turn. While Marcos was still in trance, he was able to see that both Sharon and her son Brian were *Attached.* Robert had felt a presence on Brian when they were introduced. Additionally, Brian seemed so morose and dark for a young man of twenty-two. Robert explained the situation to both Sharon and Brian and recommended that they make an appointment to see the team for a removal at their office. Robert immediately saw a look of fear on Brian's face so he reassured him everything was going to be okay. He told them the soonest the next available appointment was on Thursday. That was just two days away but Robert knew it was going to be a long two days for Brian to continue to live with those *Attachments.*

The hour arrived and everyone who was needed for the removal was present. Robert realized Sharon and Brian were anxious because they didn't know what to expect. He reassured them by going through the standard protocol with them, the use of hypnotic trance, the removal process, and the sealing of the aura in the Subtle Body. He also assured them that, if the Spirit Guide could find out, they too would learn what kind of influence the *Attachments* had on their lives.

Immediately Marcos went into trance to establish communication with the Spirit Guide known as Spencer. As their contact on the other side, Spencer began feeding them the information. He said that Brian was *Attached* by a heavy dark ghost. When alive, this man was a heroin addict from San Francisco who passed from an overdose back in 1973. He had since relocated to San Diego when he came upon Brian. Apparently, Brian was using heroin and Oxycontin at the time. The temptation was just too great for the ghost and it *Attached* to Brian. When this happens, it more than magnifies one's problems, it amplifies them exponentially. Some *Attachments* target a host with symptoms that would enable them to enter undetected. In the case of Brian, once inside meant that now there were two addicts in the same body. So even if Brian wanted to stop using he still had the ghost's addiction to deal with. Based upon experience, Robert feels this is a big problem those in rehab programs face. Those in recovery are most often blind to that part of the challenge and therefore, unequipped to deal with it and blame themselves for relapsing.

Spencer then tells them about Sharon. She was first *Attached* when she was nine years old. She had some abuse going on in her life and this is how the openings occurred. She was *Attached* by a sad motherly figure whose initial intention was to protect Sharon. It is noteworthy to explain here that not all ghosts have bad intentions when they *Attach*. Some believe they are helping their host. From experience, Robert finds that having two

141

different spirits in one body eventually results in incongruities and so makes it a policy to remove invading spirits when they are identified.

Spencer goes on to tell them Sharon was *Attached* by another ghost three years ago when she had deep bouts of depression. Now they were looking at three personalities in one body. This is how emotional roller coasters can happen. In such cases people often seek out psychotherapy or even drugs. These have some effect, but the remedy for conditions stemming from *Attachments* is removal.

After hearing all about them, the team was anxious to get to work and remove the *Attachments*. They began with Brian. Robert did a quick induction to help him relax and get him into a state of consciousness that would aid the team in getting the removal done. As soon as they went for the *Attachment*, Brian began convulsing. Tears were flowing and his body shook for a good two minutes. Knowing they were coming after him, the ghost was on the move. The trance state Marcos was in enabled him to sense where the *Attachment* was moving in the body. Marcos grasped it firmly with his hands and began removing the ghost through an energetic opening Brian already had in his chest area.

If you can envision an invisible taffy pulling machine that is basically what this extraction would look like. Taffy is a mixture of fat or butter and sugar which are boiled together to make a sticky and thick mass. After that mass is created, it needs to be stretched and pulled for a long period of time. In the past, it would have been done manually. These days, a special taffy machine is used to pull it. The machine has three bars, which spin around, pulling the taffy candy. Without the machine, the process takes a lot of effort and time. In the case of this *Attachment* removal, Marcos had to manually pull, stretch, and fold back the entity back into itself for a period of time until it was of the constitution where he could then remove it. As a result, about ten minutes passed during the which the ghost was manipulated and then removed. It was handed off to transition so that it no longer had the ability to *Attach* to anyone else.

Then it was aura sealer Daniel's turn to close the aura opening in the Subtle Body so that no other wayward ghosts could *Attach* that way in the future. He was careful to check for and close all openings from head to toe. It took no longer than ten minutes. Then Robert slowly brought Brian back to full waking consciousness. Upon opening his eyes, Robert saw an immediate transformation in Brian. Robert found himself looking at a youthful, smiling Brian. His lightness of being had returned. Robert recognized this as a turning point in which the healing could now begin. By no means was he out of the woods yet regarding his own recovery, but now Brian could address it unencumbered by the *Attachment's* influence and drain on him. In these regards, Robert knows there is a brighter light at the end of the tunnel for those like Brian who are already challenged with their own addictive behaviors.

Next, it was Sharon's turn for the removal. She at first wondered if she could even be hypnotized since she had tried before with another hypnotist and it didn't work. But within one minute of Robert's induction, she was in a deep trance. Unlike Brian's *Attachment,* those on Sharon offered little resistance as Marcos cleared her of them. Within seven minutes the removal was complete. Just as in Brian's case, Daniel now sealed Sharon's aura to complete the task. Robert returned Sharon to a state of full consciousness. When she opened her eyes, Sharon looked somewhat bewildered because she did not realize that she had been hypnotized at all. Robert let her know that the proccss was complete and that she was clear of *Attachments.* Robert noticed Sharon's appearance had a fresh, younger quality about it in comparison to when she entered his office that day.

Robert concluded the session that day by advising both Sharon and Brian to pay close attention to any changes they notice, even the subtle ones. And, to contact him again if they notice anything unusual.

Robert followed up a week later with Sharon. She told him that, since the removal, she had not cried once. Before, she confided, she cried every day. Sharon also mentioned that she noticed some big changes in her son Brian. He was more confident since the removal. She observed that he was more able to express himself much better in group situations. Overall, Sharon was very positive about her experience and went on about how she thought

Robert and his team could positively affect the lives of many more people. Robert agreed with her on that but said that he has learned that it isn't so easy getting past all of the skepticism they encounter. "We live in a world where scientific proof is needed for our minds to believe. A lot of what we deal with is of a spiritual nature. There are more people than you might first imagine that are open to such things. They are just discrete about being receptive to our work. I'm grateful for the times we are able to help people when we can.", says Robert.

The Ghost Removers never know where a case will lead them. This scenario involved more and more people and places as time went on. Robert and his team followed the leads as they came up and brought each to a successful conclusion. When all said and done, this case unfolded over a five year period.

CHAPTER 10:
WRONG PLACE, WRONG TIME

Ghosts that desire to interact or even *Attach* to living people seek out locations where they are most likely to be successful. With the increased human population, more and more facilities are being built that service the needs of the people. Some are individual structures, others are connecting hubs in a network as in the case of airport for example. But more than people and their luggage are transported from place to place. With the advent of global travel, the last five centuries have seen more new diseases than ever before become potential pandemics. Travel is also discontinuous, often including many stops and layovers along the way. This means that travelers are part of the dynamic global process of spreading infectious diseases.

But diseases are not the only hazards that are passed along these networks. These hubs are places ghosts that want to interact with living human beings are attracted to. They are target rich environments for ghosts who lay in waiting for a victim to happen along.

CASE FILE: The Hapless Tourist

Ghosts are known to congregate where people do. In this Ghost Remover case, the client, an independent contractor in his 40's, had previously successfully traveled throughout the world. To this day, he orchestrates his caseload so that he can travel unencumbered for a month at a time. He tells Robert:

> "I mapped out my travel plans for an upcoming trip to the Ukraine in my usual fashion. I did not have any thought or intention to go to Turkey. But, while in the Ukraine, I could not squelch the urge to drop everything and go to Turkey. I found myself booking a five day flight to Turkey. I left everything at my hotel and went to the airport without any baggage. After arriving in Turkey I spent five days with local people I met along the way. Then, I took a cab back to the airport and resumed my original travel plans in the Ukraine.
>
> Recognizing that this behavior was far out of character for me, I phoned Robert. Robert happened to be in session at the time. I learned through Robert that Ghost Remover Marcos, who was in the office with Robert at the time, picked up on that whoever was on the other end of that phone with Robert was *Attached* and told him so. Since I was that person on the phone, Robert informed me I was *Attached* and needed to make an appointment for a removal after I returned to San Diego, which I did.
>
> During the session with Marcos and Robert, Marcos described the *Attachment* to me as a ghost

who hung out at the airport. The ghost wanted to experience going to Turkey. The ghost identified me as a candidate to take him there so that he could have the experience through me. Marcos cleared me of this *Attachment*.

Every day people go to places that function to serve a need they have at the time. Ghosts seek out places where people with specific qualities are likely to be found to fulfill their specific goals. For instance, a ghost who wants to experience acting may haunt a theater and so forth.

In the case of the Hapless Tourist, on the surface, it appears that he merely took an abrupt and unexpected detour which resulted in a totally unexpected strange new adventure. When in reality, like a puppet master animating a puppet connected by strings to a handle from which it can be manipulated, the *Attachment* took the Hapless tourist on a detour from his destination in the Ukraine to Turkey instead. This client later reports that never before, or since the clearing has he ever abruptly changed course in such a manner during any other trip.

But one may ask the question here, "If an *Attachment* can make a tourist drop everything and fly to another country on an unexpected adventure, what else are they capable of?"

Airports are not the only places teeming with people and activity on a consistent basis. Humans have created other hubs that serve many different purposes for humans as well as ghosts. This next case is an example of what can happen when a person is in the wrong place at the wrong time.

148

Immigration is the international movement of people into a destination country of which they are not natives or where they do not possess citizenship in order to settle or reside there.

Illegal immigration into the United States has been a hotly debated topic in recent times. It refers to the migration of people into a country in ways that violate the immigration laws of that country, or the remaining in a country of people who no longer have the legal right to remain.

Stopping illegal immigration starts at the border. However, it continues inside the United States as well. The United States Border Patrol operates traffic checkpoints near the Mexico-United States border to deter illegal immigration and smuggling activities.

Up next, **CASE FILE:** The Case of An Immigrant's Dilemma.

Robert: In this situation I had a hunch that this woman could have an *Attachment* as a result of the situation she had been thrown into. In those kind of situations we know Attachments would linger in a place like that because either weakened people would come into the ICE facility or in time people in custody would become weakened and thereby vulnerable to becoming *Attached*. Weakness could stem from mental, emotional, or physical trauma, depression, environmental issues and so forth. One or more ghosting spirits of the dead could *Attach* to a person in that facility. I inquired with our spirit guide as to whether or not client (E) was *Attached* and the response was that she did get *Attached*. Therefore she is here today to learn about the *Attachments* and for a removal of them. Before we proceed, here is her story.

Evelyn: I am a best-selling author who entered the United States legally on a journalist VISA.

A VISA is a conditional authorization granted by a country to a foreigner, allowing them to enter, remain within, or to leave that country. Visas typically include limits on the duration of the foreigner's stay, territory within the country they may enter, the dates they may enter, the number of permitted visits or an individual's right to work in the country in question. A VISA can be revoked at any time.

Prior to this incident I had consulted an immigration attorney prior to the VISA expiration date and was assured that everything was okay during the renewal process as long as I remained inside the United States. So, I felt confident that my papers were in order and that I had nothing to fear.

I am a bestselling author. In September of 2018 I was invited to speak at a 3-day festival being held in the mountains in Southeast San Diego. I knew that this place was inside the territory of the United States. Returning from that festival we drove through an Immigration and

Customs Enforcement (ICE) checkpoint. The officers asked "Is everybody a US citizen here?" Confident that my VISA was in order I raised my hand and said, "No". "I'm from Poland." After checking my papers I was immediately detained by immigration and customs enforcement also known as ICE. My first concern was for my son. Upon being taken into custody my friends in the car said that they would see to my son.

I was arrested and then put into a border patrol car. From there I was taken to a holding station where I remained for six days and nights. While there, I was under fluorescent lights 24/7. At night, I slept on the floor under an aluminum blanket.

Interned with me were women from all over the world in all stages of life. There were pregnant women, mothers with children, and seniors. Men were held in another cell but I could see them as they would be taken in and out of their cell. Some were tired from the transport through the desert by Coyotes. Some were visibly injured. Lots of people had trauma and shock from being away from their home. Some were poor people. Others had criminal records.

During the six day stay I was refusing food because my diet is normally very healthy, very pure with lots of organic fruits and vegetables with intermittent periods of fasting. As a result, I didn't feel that a diet consisting of burritos and Kool-Aid was nutritional food. I gave it to other people who appeared to be hungry. In keeping with past experiences of fasting, during my six day fast, I was finding my mind very clear and had a lot of energy. I felt like my own light was very strong which was a bit too strong for such a dark place.

I am a European English speaking Caucasian journalist and aware of my rights and so I had a sense that I was safe even under this type of detention. Whereas I could not assure others there that everything would be alright for them.

After six days in the ICE holding station at the San Ysidro border I was transferred to one of the worst ICE prisons in America located in the United States near the Mexican border. It is run by CoreCivic, formerly the Corrections Corporation of America (CCA), is a company that owns and manages private prisons and detention centers and operates others on a concession basis. I was kept there for six weeks.

Emotional traumas ran high. I witnessed a lot of suffering there. There is the pain of mother's being separated from their children. I was separated from my son. However, unlike most other women there, I knew my son was okay and being taken care of by friends who have other children.

I witnessed many people requiring medical care who were not getting any. Medical care available was at the most basic level.

For example, I saw women with broken bones given Advil for the pain and bandaids for their injuries. There were no x-rays. Nurses advised patients to shut-up and not complain.

As with the first ICE facility, the quality of food at this prison was very bad. At this point I realized that I cannot continue fasting. By this time I was coming to the realization that my belief that my situation would be quickly sorted out was inaccurate. Officials at this facility asked me on multiple occasions what I was doing there. I assume they asked because I was Caucasian. To which I replied, You made a mistake. You let a journalist in here who has seen what is going on in here behind your iron gates.

In the same way as the first holding station, quality of food at this ICE prison lacked nutrition. They don't feed people properly. I first noticed that right after eating the food that I was off. I couldn't go to the bathroom. I became constipated and was in pain. I didn't defecate for five days. Many other women were experiencing this. I inquired about fruits and vegetables but these were denied. Therefore, I requested laxatives to relieve the bloating but it did not helped. Eventually, I was able to purchase pico and Raman at a kiosk but that too was bad. However, my abdomen remained inflamed and swollen and I'm even experiencing this still, even now.

I experienced brain fog. I did not have mental clarity. It was impossible to sleep normally because I was under fluorescent lights 24/7. My eyesight was affected and my eyes became sensitive to light. There were sounds coming from so many people. Radios, walkee talkees and the like. As a result I experienced sleep deprivation.

And the entire time I knew that my situation was different. I knew that I was safe because my skin color protected me. I speak English. I know my rights. However, I really felt for the people that were going through all of this.

However, while I was held there, I had some of the most beautiful and meaningful conversations with other detainees that I've ever had in my life. I experienced sisterhood with women from other countries. During my ten years in America I never felt this kind of connection with the people. There was a real sense of humanity amongst the detainees.

After my release from the ICE prison, I found it very difficult to deal with the natural daylight and everyday noises. It was almost like PTSD symptoms. Even weeks afterwards, my eyes are still hurting. I continue to experience brain fog. I don't have mental clarity. My abdomen is inflamed and swollen. I feel like I need a lot of healing to recover from these symptoms.

Robert: Now we are going to prepare for the removal

Antoinette will go into a hypnotic trance. Then, spirit guide Lane will come in. He can detail where the *Attachments* are located in Evelyn and provide other information that becomes available during session.

Lane: Wow! That is an amazing story. I am sorry that you went through that. The separation from your child is what caused your vulnerability to becoming *Attached*. There are fourteen *Attachments*. They all came on at the same time. These entities were originally *Attached* to other people in the facility. There are many men and women in there who are *Attached*. It is a sad situation. Although, you did bring some light and laughter to some of the folks you interacted with. These *Attachments* are making you feel uneasy now. They are adversely exasperating your symptoms and making it so that you don't feel good, even now. I will be taking them off. After I do, it may take up to three days for you to have a sense of feeling back to normal again. However, the effects on your eyesight and sensitivity to light now is from the time you were exposed to the fluorescent lights. There is some weight gain as a result of your body storing food but that too will level out soon.

I will be removing the entities. They are residing in your entire body. However, I will pull them out through your navel area because that was the entrance point. I will pull everything out from there. Afterwards, I will seal the opening in that area that allowed them to enter in the first place.

To me, their presence in your entire body gives you a sense of feeling consumed or being eaten alive.

Evelyn: Yes. Even though I have been taking care of myself since being released, I still experience the symptoms.

Robert: I'm placing Evelyn in a light trance for this *Attachment* removal.

(Antoinette/Lane position themselves for the removal.)

Lane: There are fourteen really bad *Attachments*. These *Attachments* are vocal. They are people who have died in custody inside the ICE detention center where Evelyn was being held. They wanted to get a 'ride' or way out because they were trapped in the place by other *Attachments* and entities in the vicinity. They needed to *Attach* to Evelyn so that they could depart the facility when she was released.

They do want to transition which is good. They are going to the other side happily. They convey their gratitude and are saying thank you. Upon departing, one ghost has given me her name, Isabelle. I'm acknowledging her. These ghosts are expressing to me that they died there.

Evelyn: That's quite possible given the conditions and lack of medical care there.

Lane: Seems to me like some things that are occurring in the ICE facility needs to be exposed to others.

(Note: Eveylyn's stomach begins to gurgle loudly as they exit her abdomen.

Lane: Now I'm doing an energetic type cleaning of the abdominal area. Now that the entities are gone, I'm sealing up the opening. Please remain where you are until I complete this process.

(After completing the process, Antoinette/Lane return to their seat.)
Lane: The only remaining part of this story is in regards to Isabelle. Isabelle was one of fourteen *Attachments*. She asked me if there was a way to help the other people that are ghosting inside the ICE facility.

Robert: Can we do that with our other spirit guide Pacer?

Lane: Unfortunately, we cannot do that. There are ghosts and *Attachments* being held prisoners there by other 'bad' ghosts and *Attachments* who are holding up any other ghost who would like to go or transition. So that situation will make it hard for us to clear the area. Given the situation there, the only means for these fourteen *Attachments* to get out from under the dark entities that were holding them in place there was to *Attach* to Evelyn and leave with here when she was released.

Isabelle is now conveying that she only wanted help. Another of our spirit guides named Priscilla helped Isabelle crossover. Isabelle is happy now that she crossed over. I'm being told that these fourteen spirits will now have access to their own spirit guides. In time, they will be able to regroup on the other side in the spirit realm.

Lane: In regards to post removal guidance, Evelyn, I realize that you already know how to take care of yourself and how to eat well so I don't need to talk about that. I suggest that you add meditation into your wellness program. Twenty minutes nightly should be good for you. The move you are contemplating to Asia seems to me like it would be good for you.

Evelyn: I plan on writing a book about my experience to help people become aware of what goes on in the detention facility and shed new light on the spiritual aspect of what happened to me in regards to these *Attachments*.

As a follow-up to Evelyn's case, spirit guide Lane checked on her son, though emotionally traumatized as a result of the separation from his mother, he is not *Attached*.

Fourteen spirits of the dead had *Attached* to the Evelyn as a means of escaping the hierarchy they described as imprisoning them in their web. In other words, they couldn't escape the clutches of the dark entities that held them nor could they leave the facility until they *Attached* to a human host who subsequently walked out of the building and off the premises. The Ghost Remover freed the woman of these 14 *Attachments* and aided the spirits in transitioning. However, the dark hierarchy remains in place at the immigration detention facility and continues to terrorize and control other spirits in the vicinity. The unseen effects of the dark entities can take many forms. This case is an example of one of them.

As a result of this case, we can begin to contemplate the adverse effects of detention center conditions, separations of family members, quality of food, 24-hour artificial fluorescent lights, and unreported deaths in the facility on the people incarcerated because these conditions weaken their vitality.

Ghosts of a specific nature or interest will be drawn to one type of facility or another. For instance some ghosts may be attracted to airports whereas others are drawn to prisons.

Within the walls of modern prisons, many troubled dysfunctional people are warehoused in tight quarters against their will. Sentences vary. Some even have life sentences. For those on death row, the possibility of execution awaits them. All of their emotions, along with those of the armed guards who are posted to watch them continuously, converge upon one another.

As these people live, eat, sleep and breathe together day after day, in such confinement, their individual energy fields (aka Subtle Bodies) generate a group energy field. Referred to as morphogenetic fields,[10] the ones that surround a prison could best be described as 'dark'. Ghosts can see these energies clearly. Some ghosts would avoid such places while others would be drawn to them.

Prisons and detention centers are targets for spirits of a darkened nature that seek to either haunt or *Attach*. Being oblivious to *Attachments,* the incarceration system is, out of ignorance, housing both victims and victimizers. Incarcerated prisoners are often reputed to have troubled childhoods. Their personal histories increase the odds of having become vulnerable to *Attachments*. If they are not already *Attached* before they enter the prison system, it is more than likely that they are by the time they leave the place. As a result of being confined and all that goes with that experience, prisoners are disadvantaged in their ability to maintain the state of health and well-being that could otherwise deter a ghost from targeting them. If *Attached* at the time of their release from jail, their issues are then compounded by the *Attachment* while they are attempting to rehabilitate and reestablish themselves. Instead of an old-fashioned ball-and-chain that weighted prisoners down so that they could not travel far, *Attachments* are in effect, a ball-and-chain of a different kind. As with anything, changes begin with awareness.

---

[10] Suggested Resource: Morphic Resonance: The Nature of Formative Causation by Rupert Sheldrake.

According to The Washington Post, "Though only five percent of the world's population lives in the United States, it is home to twenty-five percent of the world's prison population."[11] This is a disturbing statistic. Are more people getting incarcerated in the United States because we have more 'bad' people? Or, is it possible that more people have become *Attached*? If these *Attachments* have criminal tendencies themselves, they would be attracted to *Attach* to those that have the potential to commit crimes, exerting influence in that direction. This could result in the crime and incarceration rates increasing.

---

[11] Source: https://www.washingtonpost.com/...does-the-united... (April 30, 2015)

CHAPTER 11:
MORE UNIQUE CASES

In this next case of unfinished business, the re-connection is sought not for an apology (as was the case in Chapter 2), but for a personal vendetta involved. In those cases, vengeance is sought by the entities no matter where it leads to. They want a kind of retaliation designed to extract retribution to balance the scales of justice because someone feels wronged as in the following example.

CASE FILE: Ancient Scottish Warriors
Robert writes:

> Having heard about us, a family of four travelled to San Diego from Houston, Texas on the 4th of July weekend. After checking them, we learned this whole family was *Attached*. We were astonished to discover at the removal that these ghosts were seeking revenge and had been searching for this husband for over three thousand years. During the session, spirit guides told us that this man lived in Scotland in a previous life during the Beaker period and took part in the slaughter of an entire village. Women, children, everyone in the village was killed. These murdered Scottish warrior ghosts finally found him in this life and *Attached* to his entire

family causing all kinds of issues in an effort to destroy his family just as he had destroyed theirs so long ago. We cleared this family of thirty *Attachments* confident the spirit guides would transition them to their next place in the afterlife.

Vendettas are quite common. There seems to be no end to the types of grudges one person holds against another that they carry with them into the next life. It seems logical to conclude that forgiveness plays an important role in releasing oneself and others from hard feelings that carry on well after the people have expired. Beyond that, Robert says: "I find cases like Ancient Scottish Warriors fascinating because I hear about historical events and time periods I am completely unfamiliar with during these sessions. This happens a lot. In this case, I wondered about the Beaker period. A Google search resulted in a lot of information about the people and the times."

Mainly, the name, "Beaker People" is derived from the vessels they drank from and buried with the dead. They date as far back as 2500 BCE. The influx of this extraordinary people, with their superior technologies, is believed to have been largely peaceful, but their capabilities inevitably allowed them to dominate the existing population wherever they settled. They are recognized as the ones who introduced metalwork to Scotland. Scottish culture was changed dramatically by their arrival and the advent of metalworking.

But if Robert and his team had not cleared the Texas family of the *Attachments,* in all likelihood, they would have remained *Attached* until their own deaths. It may also give the appearance that the *Attachments* 'died' with them, but that isn't necessarily true.

For example, there has been only one removal done on a client where it was discovered that she was born into this life while *Attached* by a ghost who was *Attached* to her from a past life. Robert says, "Based on experience, it appears that it is highly unlikely that an *Attachment* would remain *Attached* to a human host after the death of that person. Instead, upon the death of the living person, the *Attachment* finds another living host."

According to Robert, "The longest an *Attachment* we've cleared had been *Attaching* to new subsequent living human hosts, one after another, after each person's passing was 500 years. Over five centuries, it body hopped from one victim to the next until we finally turned it over to its spirit guide who transitioned it to the afterlife."

One can see how the *Attachment* population continues to grow at rates unsurpassed in human history because many of those that exist are not departing. Likewise, the number of ghosts that have previous *Attachment* experiences is increasing as well. This means that there are more of the severest and most dangerous ones among us than ever before.

Robert previously explained the scenario this way. "*Attachments* consider removal a kind of death. It is because they didn't transition to the afterlife at death, they are afraid of moving on and therefore see it as the death they never had to experience. But in fact, their spirit guides are waiting for them as they have been all along to help them transition."

CASE FILE: More than a real estate transaction.

People around the world experience moving from one residence into another. For example, Americans move on average twelve times during their lifetime. One couple purchased a new home in the Laguna Hills area of Orange County in Southern California near Laguna Beach. However, in this case, they got more than they bargained for.

In August of 2018 Robert received a phone call from a new home owner who reported paranormal activity in the house. He described his attempts to shift the energy and had a complete remodel underway at the time. His wife was so creeped out by the ghost activity that she would not stay there until her husband found the means to clear the place. He conveyed that he was not as affected by the ghosts as his wife. In fact, he was skeptical. But given the nature of the situation, he felt he had no other recourse but to call Robert for help.

He was adamant that he did must remain anonymous. And, that he did not any of the remodel crew to become aware that Robert and Antoinette were there to do a Ghost Removal. Upon arriving, he ushered Robert and Antoinette in quickly. They wasted no time. Robert placed Antoinette in trance. Her spirit guide described many ghosts in the Laguna Beach area that were from the indigenous peoples that inhabited the area in the not too distant past. Antoinette described and communicated with one female ghost who had come into the residence and been the one responsible for the paranormal activity. She had taken an interest in the man and was toying with the wife through paranormal activity. He didn't seem interested in the details and urged Antoinette to proceed.

The ghosts in the area described a sense of irritation of being 'walked through' by living human beings in the highly populated beach areas. Consequently, some have moved into the Laguna Hills area to reduce the incidences of close encounters with the living. Because the ghosts in the vicinity were not bothering the residents and did not want to transition, the spirit guide created an energetic type of protection bubble around the home so that they would avoid it in the future. Next, the ghost that had intruded and who was responsible for the paranormal activity was ready to transition and did so. The homeowner promptly ushered Robert and Antoinette out of the house.

On the ride home Antoinette described the female ghost as she appeared to her in her native attire. The ghost described herself as having been a Female Chief of the Tongva tribe.

Afterwards, an internet search of Wikipedia revealed that the Tongva are a Native American people of Southern California. Along with the neighboring Chumash, the Tongva were the most powerful indigenous people to inhabit Southern California. At the time of European contact, they may have numbered between five and ten thousand people. Additionally, they are reputed to have had female chiefs.

In this case, the new homeowners purchased their new home and got more than they bargained for. Their home included a ghost. Americans move on average twelve times during their lifetime. It is possible therefore, that in at least one of those homes had additional occupants in the form of ghosts. Likewise, people around the globe are probably interacting with spirits of the dead all the time. They just don't know it.

It is the combination of the human population explosion and high rates of trauma combined with self-destructive coping mechanisms that results in increased weakness and vulnerability in populations all over the globe. This combination has created the 'perfect storm'. Opportunities for ghosting spirits that want to *Attach* have never been more bountiful.

Sometimes while they are communicating with the spirit realm, the Ghost Removers get directed into a completely unexpected direction. For instance, in 2009, while their necromancer was already in a hypnotic trance to do other spirit communication, Robert thought to make an inquiry about a missing person in the San Diego area named Amber Dubois. He wrote down the information relayed through the medium and mailed it to the tip hotline set up by the authorities for people to report any leads they might have on the case. Robert knew the information might not be well received since their reading indicated Amber was deceased.

Amber's mother, Carrie, later told Robert that she had received many readings through the hot line. She did not want to believe her daughter Amber was dead and so ignored any readings that might indicate that. However, some time afterwards, during the trial of the accused murderer, she read the account Robert sent to her. It was the closest to the actual information that had been discovered over the course of the investigation. So, after the trial, she contacted him. They spoke on the phone. Robert invited Carrie to a session with the necromancer so that she would have an opportunity to communicate with Amber. She accepted. Afterwards, Carrie said she felt like she had gotten closure that she desperately needed that day. Despite all that happened, after communicating with her, she now felt Amber was indeed, okay.

Since that time, Carrie has gone on to create a foundation that helps the parents of missing children called Amber Rescue. She contacts Robert on certain cases to communicate through the necromancer for information the spirit world might have that could shed some light on an unsolved case and bring resolution to the family. She has done some incredible work and had some remarkable encounters as evidenced in this next case involving her dog.

Over time, Robert and his team have experienced all kinds of different spirit communications. They have found that animals, especially pets like dogs and cats, can see ghosts as well as *Attachments*. The dogs themselves revealed that they may seem to adversely react to someone, even strike out at a person when in fact, they are responding to the *Attachment,* not the person. When the Ghost Remover team works on location, they are often accompanied by their animal communicator just in case it is possible to receive information about a case from an animal resource. But in this next case, the dog was the conduit which led to an amazing event.

CASE FILE: The Spirit Guided Canine
Robert recalls, "In 2011, two and a half years after her daughter died, Carrie was helping in the search for missing nursing student Michelle Le in Northern California near Alameda County Park. At that time Carrie had her one-year-old yellow

Labrador named Amber, in her daughter's memory, with her. Carrie told me that she never intended to take the animal on a search that day, but she's grateful she changed her mind."

"Carrie later told me that after taking the animal's leash off, Amber the dog bolted down a trail and out of sight. She called several times for her dog to return to her but she did not. Carrie thought that she must have been following a search group that was deployed earlier. She went after the dog. Moments later, she spotted her dog who had stopped in a flat area."

"When she reached the spot the dog was located at she bent down to re-attach her leash to the collar when she noticed what could possibly be some sort of remains. She returned to the group and alerted an officer on the team. Even though Amber the dog was very young and not trained as a cadaver dog, Carrie was impressed by her drive and natural ability to search. She felt her dog was truly a hero."

"I have to believe it was Amber and Michelle guiding her. There's no real explanation for what she did. I have a tremendous amount of sadness not only reliving my own tragedy, but also for the Le family," Carrie explained to the press.[12]

---

[12] References for this account was obtained from CBS8.com at:http://www.cbs8.com/story/15519582/amazing-story-of-how-ambers-mom-found-michelle-les-body Posted: Sep 21, 2011 5:03pm PDT.

"It's a great pleasure to be able to serve another family to bring some kind of closure to that family. I feel it's made me a stronger person." she added. "I know that God, my daughter Amber, and Michelle needed me. This is my job. This is what I was supposed to do with my life." McGonigle said.

Robert Major had been following Carrie's new found passion in the organization called Amber Rescue that she championed after the murder of her daughter. Carrie works resources and personally goes out to find missing girls in similar situations as her daughters. Robert and his team had worked with Carrie on two cases in which the deceased victims were communicated with via the team's Necromancer in an effort to obtain other information that might help the living resolve the case.

Robert continues, "I was quite intrigued when I read in the newspaper that Carrie was responsible for finding the body of Michelle Le. I knew that her dog was only about a year old and untrained. I was curious how the dog found the body later identified as Michelle. So, I phoned Carrie and invited her and the dog to come to the house to learn more from the dog through our animal communicator. Carrie brought both of her dogs because she also wanted to communicate with the older dog."

"I had assembled members of our team for the meeting which included our animal communicator and Necromancer." says Robert. "During the session it became evident that the young dog really had very little to do with the finding of the body according to Carrie's deceased daughter Amber, who communicated through the Necromancer. She told us that *she* had guided the dog to Michelle's body because she wanted her mom to get credit for all the work that she's doing through Amber Rescue."

"Carrie told me that the dog had broken free from her grasp and ran some three hundred yards to an area that had already been searched by the police search and rescue. The dog went over and sat down where the body was and wouldn't move.", says Robert. "Carrie of course, went to retrieve the dog and that is when she noticed the body. She went and told authorities which is how she was given the credit for her work that her deceased daughter Amber wanted her to have."

Robert and his team have occasionally assisted on missing persons cases. However when it involves a death, their Necromancer senses the experience of the death which can be traumatic and painful for him. Therefore, it is not something they normally pursue.

Humans are not the only species that can end up ghosting. Animals can too. Like human ghosts, they too can disrupt the living but can they *Attach?*. By now Robert had thought he'd seen it all but this next story had elements to it that even shocked Robert.

CASE FILE: Wild Child

A family from the Northwest area of the United States had contacted Robert to inquire whether or not their 'wild' six year old son was *Attached*. After checking, Robert conveyed to John that his son was indeed *Attached*. It took the family a few months to arrange a trip to the San Diego area for a removal. Eventually, they drove the twelve hours to San Diego.

John had described his son's behavior as 'wild' to Robert but he did not suspect that he was truly 'wild'. Upon their arrival at the Ghost Remover office expressed that he was determined not to have anything to do with Robert or Antoinette. .

 Little did he suspect that the son was truly 'wild'. The boy promptly left the office located on the second floor and walked along the balcony. As he did this, he said that he wasn't coming it. After quite a bit of coaxing, bribes, and threats from both parents, he reluctantly came back into the office.

Robert placed Antoinette in trance so that she could communicate with her spirit guide Lane. They learned that the boy had eight *Attachments* on him. Four were native Americans. However, the other four were large felines, leopards. The Ghost Removers had never encountered this in the eighteen years they had been doing *Attachment* removals.

During the assessment process, the boy moved on all fours crawling under chairs and behind the desk. From there, he jumped up and down from the massage table in the office for clients to lay upon during removals. Next, he went under the massage table. From there, he stared up at Robert and growled like a large cat. Robert later explained that he could see the fear in the boys eyes.

Robert next inquired with spirit guide Lane as to how the boy was *Attached* by the leopards. He replied: "The Indians are telling me that they brought them in when he was just an infant." Robert was relieved to learn that the leopards had not *Attached* to the boy on their own accord. He thought he'd seen it all over the years and was glad to know that this was not something he would likely encounter in the future.

The next step in the process was to clear the boy of these *Attachments*. To do that, they needed him to remain stable but he wouldn't lie still long enough for the entire pieces. Antoinette and her spirit guides got bits and pieces as best they could. Finally, they were able to capture and remove the lead leopard. After that, the boy settled down enough to where they could clear him completely.

Immediately after being cleared, the boy calms down and begins talking as if nothing had just transpired. He appeared to everyone in the room as a young boy having a conversation with the people in the room. His mother then looked and Robert and said, "When he was two and a half he told me he was the Mom and he was the boss." After hearing the *Attachment* assessment, correlating the 'wild' behavior to the leopards, and now seeing her son behaving normally after the removal, she realized that it was the leopard talking to her at that time and not her son.

As with other cases, often times other family members are also *Attached*. This case was no different. Because of the area in the Northwest they reside in, they were all *Attached* by Native American ghosts. In this case, they expressed a belief that it was okay to disrupt the white people in this way as retribution for having had their lives cut short. They had a desire to be here on earth and live their lives out in any capacity they could even if it meant it was at this families expense. Antoinette and her spirit guides cleared everyone else with no problem. Both the Native Americans and the leopards successfully transition to the afterlife.

Prior to closing the session, spirit guide Lane told the boy's parents that he will most likely still have residual behaviors which should pass in the next two to three months.

Robert always follows up with clients. In this case, John contacted Robert with this update. "My son is making huge strides. He feels to me to be more like himself. Prior to the removal, he could barely talk coherently. Now, we're having some mature conversations. The younger siblings are still fearful of him. They don't understand that he's different now that he's cleared. My wife and I notice that the wild look that would come over his eyes no longer happens. The look in his eyes are consistently normal.

But, as a result of past experiences with our son, the other children tend to treat him like he is still *Attached* even though he is behaving so much nicer to them now. We are patient because we see the recovery from this as a process. Thanks to you we are starting afresh. It'll take time for our son to build trust with his siblings. We are very thankful.

With the benefit of hindsight, it now appears to the boy's parents that, in some instances, the leopards were, at times, in possession of their son's body.

The term for a complete take-over is *extreme possession* and is described as follows. In the extreme form of possession the abnormal personality of the invading spirit replaces the normal personality of the host completely. The victim fully identifies himself as the *Invading Spirit.*[13]

Attachment is one thing but *extreme possession* is an insidious type of *Identity Theft.* Only it is your actual body that is stolen for a time while *you* are usurped. *You* become either a helpless bystander or are totally unaware that another spirit has taken control of your body and is, by virtue of their physical appearance, impersonating *You!*

Extreme possession victims may not understand that they are the victim of this type of *Identity Theft* because most modern societies do not acknowledge that it exists. As a result, victims are often bewildered and frustrated. And, without credibility, with the exception Robert and his team, they are left with nowhere to turn for help.

Unfortunately for some, *extreme possession* can have deadly consequences.

CASE FILE: Saratoga Springs, NY
In October of 2013 Robert learned about a murder, suicide involving two people who were his long time friends that

---

[13] Source: By the Finger of God by S. Vernon McCasland

lived in New York.

Robert had known John and Patricia for years. John had wanted a break from the family restaurant and bar near the Saratoga racetrack so he moved to San Diego where he met Robert. Through John, Robert met his mother Patricia. They got along well and the next time Robert was in New York, he visited Patricia at her place of business, the Bayshores Tropic Hut and Marina.

According to Robert, after four or five years John eventually moved back to New York to work in the family business again. While living there, he had a very nice girlfriend. Robert describes John as having been well-liked and popular amongst many mutual friends. However, during the year prior to the incident, Robert heard from his friend Tony who lives in New York that John's girlfriend had left him. John's life seemed to have taken an abrupt downward spiral. Tony described John as appearing uncharacteristically haggard and gaunt.

In the weeks that followed, Robert received the news of their murder suicide. The following gruesome account is from the October 2013 Times Union newspaper.

> John stabbed his mother to death and then spent half a day with her body before shooting himself, Saratoga Springs police said Saturday.
>
> John, 47, and his mother, Patricia, 75, were

found in their Union Avenue mobile home next to Bayshores Tropic Hut Friday by a family friend who hadn't heard from them in days.

Police said that on Monday, John assaulted his mother, breaking several of her bones, and then stabbed her to death. John then remained in the mobile home for 12 to 14 hours before shooting and killing himself in the late afternoon. ...

Some who work in the area said the pair had been seen yelling at each other on numerous occasions. On Friday, one man who declined to give his name and was a bar patron said he had seen the volatile relationship between mother and son, but he was shocked to hear of the deaths.

For Robert, learning about the deaths was a shock. Knowing them both personally, he decided to check with the spirit world to find out if he could learn more about what happened. The spirit guide explained to Robert that both mother and son were *Attached*. The Spirit Guide indicated that the *Attachments* did not like each other nor did they get along. *Their* arguing escalated. By all outward appearances, it seemed as though it was John and Patricia who were arguing but it was the *Attachments* that were arguing with each other. The *Attachments* were growing in strength and intensity, at times, possessing each of the hosts. When they were '*In*', they fought with each other but it appeared to everyone else that it was John and Patricia who were arguing. Not all *Attachments* can possess a living human being, argue, fight, and commit a heinous criminal act; but some can, and some do.

Apparently, the *Attachment* that possessed John killed Patricia. The Spirit Guide who checked on the situation indicated that the *Attachments* had a significant role in this murder suicide. This is not to imply that all criminals are possessed when they commit crimes. Nor that all *Attachments* can drive a living human being to commit a criminal act. But some can.

Robert recalled several other cases that he was aware of in which the *Attachment* possessed a person and committed murder. He states that it is more common that one would think.

After checking on them, Robert discovered that neither John nor Patricia is ghosting. However, anyone can get lost in the transition to the afterlife.

But more than likely, the ghosts that had *Attached* to John and Patricia hopped off rather than die with the host body. In turn, the more experience an entity garners makes them serial offenders and therefore more dangerous and problematic for the living after each and every successful takeover. They can quickly advance in. In some case, they take-over completely.

They may wait until they become strong enough themselves or bring in others and gain strength through numbers. They often recruit weaker ghosts who are in alignment with their character as allies to support their mission to collapse the host's spirit and achieve their impending takeover. In the case of multiple *Attachments,* the

Attachments that are aware of others often will struggle to unseat and displace one another as each vies for a larger fragment of a life. As a result of the duress and stress, the original host may leave their own body to the *Attachments* who then fight it out amongst themselves.

Ghosts also tend to pool together. Some gather in like-minded groups waiting for an opportunity to act out on whatever was left undone. Just as a strong or charismatic personality that can gather living people into groups and influence them, a strong spirit can do the same. These kindred spirits are often seen in severe *Attachment* cases where one strong entity has gathered others to try and influence, haunt and even step '*In*' and take over the host to reenact or act out their own vendettas on those it deems the enemy. In some cases that can manifest into other military conflicts.

Even in extreme possession cases where one or more *Attachments* succeed in defeating the host spirit, if everything has gone well, the human body they intend to inhabit is still intact and they can begin to function immediately. But there is no 'happily ever after' ending to this story. More often than not, the other *Attachments* that globed on over time are not all defeated and did not depart along with the host spirit. These *Attachments* continue to exert all the strategies and tactics that they have observed and learned along the way and are now part of their arsenal. As a result, instead of a serene environment in which one soul inhabits and is in command, the struggle continues. Therefore, *his* thoughts and daily life are constantly intruded upon. He too is usurped of the ability to envision a clear mental picture for his own future because of the nature of the *Attachment* cycle.

There are cases Robert and his team have come across in which the original host's spirit is gone. That spirit is no longer connected to the body he was born in. Instead, the body is solely inhabited by *Attachments*. Most often, a few (one-to-three) are generally in charge. In all of these cases so far, Robert and his team have had to respectfully decline to perform a clearing because they and their spirit helpers have not been guided to make a determination as to which *Attachment* should get the body to inhabit as their own.

CHAPTER 12:
THE GHOST REMOVERS
ON LOCATION

Throughout history humans have died in many different ways, illness, old age, accidents, murder, combat and even capital punishment to name a few. Some people consider the person is dead and gone. This is not necessarily so. They are not always 'dead' or 'gone' in the normal sense especially if they died in a violent or unexpectedly abrupt manner. Their spirit has merely left the range of our physical senses.

The initial element in the *Attachment* cycle is ghosting. Because ghosting is the first phase in the cycle, it warrants further consideration. We know from information presented earlier that Robert has found that some people get stuck because of their beliefs. One example of that was when the teenager died in the auto accident from Chapter 1. Instead of moving on, she heeded her mother's guidance which was, *"If you're ever in trouble, stay put. I will come and find you."* The young gal did as her mom instructed. She waited by the accident scene where she had been killed until Robert contacted her. Beliefs can have unintended consequences as in the case where many believe that their grave is their 'final resting place'. As a result, they don't move on.

There are many reasons people fail to make the transition. Here are accounts of others.

CASE FILE: A Family Affair (continued from Chapter 9)
To recap, this story is part of the Case File presented earlier. It occurred over a five year period. Charles had written Robert about how he wanted to speak to his grandson Taylor who had died in an automobile accident.

Robert writes:

> Charles had been so distraught looking for some type of closure. Our motto has always been "Help ease the pain." I knew Charles was in a lot of pain. I had to call in our Necromancer Sam and ask for a special favor because he was no longer active with our team. I told him that this man really needed our help. Sammy had left the team because the work became too painful. He would re-live the pains and the emotions of the people we were contacting at the time of their death and it became too much for him. He is the best there is at what he does but I could no longer see him suffer even if it meant our team losing his abilities. If I feel it's really important I will call Sam for help and this was one of those cases.
>
> It took a little convincing on my part to enlist Sam's help but once he heard Charles's story he agreed. We all met the next day at my sister Antoinette's house. It took a few moments to get Sam comfortable in trance because it had been a while since he'd been hypnotized. Once in trance, Taylor was present within about thirty seconds.

When a soul is ghosting it only takes a moment for contact to take place. Plus we're more confident that we have the right person.

Taylor was a lost soul stuck in the netherworld. All the emotional pain his family and friends were experiencing made it too hard for him to move on. Our sessions create a space so the person ghosting can say goodbye to their loved ones and proceed to move on. Taylor wanted to leave a message for his mom saying he was so sorry. He wanted her to wear the blue dress he loved so much and he wanted her to stop crying for him. There was more communication between Taylor and his grandfather Charles before we said our good-byes. Upon closing the session we ask the person ghosting if they are ready to go to the light. In most cases they go. I then brought Sam out of trance and I could see his eyes were still tearing up from all the emotions he felt. Charles was in a better place it seemed and he let us know how grateful he was. He just wished his daughter would have attended the session too.

Nearly five years had passed when I received an email from Charles asking if it might be possible for his daughter Sharon to contact Taylor. It would soon be the five-year anniversary of Taylor's death and she was having a hard time with it. She still cried every single day. I told Charles to have Sharon email me and I would make arrangements. We now have Marcos who can do what Sam used to do for the team. Sharon began writing me saying she knew Taylor was still present at the house and she wanted him to move on and could we help with that? I responded we could and that I needed her to let Taylor know we were going to meet and to be present for us. She could do that by thinking it or saying it so that Taylor could pick up on her intention. I thought she must be feeling Taylor visiting from the spirit world since he had agreed to cross over. I told her we would be at her place on the anniversary of his passing. It was late afternoon when we got there.

Wayne, Taylor's step dad greeted us and ushered us into the house passing the garden and the mini shrine that had been made for Taylor. I set up my movie camera in the living room to record the session as the rest of the family nervously found their seats. I took a few moments to explain how the process would work and did my best to put everyone at ease.

Marcos instantly entered trance which drew everyone's attention to him. I could see a smile come to his face right away as he started to speak. Taylor is present and he's been ghosting here for the entire five years. Of course I immediately ask "Taylor, I thought you had gone to the light?" (Because Taylor was ghosting but not *Attaching* he was not forced to transition previously.) Marcos said it was too difficult for him to leave his family and he decided to stay hoping he could somehow help ease their sadness and his own personal pain.

The session was full of conversation back and forth with Taylor from everyone present. There was some laughter and there were plenty of tears shed before we were done. Taylor promised to move on this time as he thanked us and expressed his love to everyone. Since the light was there for him to go to we also sent the four ghosting dogs who had passed in previous five years and fourteen other ghosts who were in the surrounding area. The place became instantly lighter once everybody had crossed.

While Marcos was still in trance he was able to see that both Sharon and Brian were *Attached* by ghosts. I had felt it right away when I met Brian. He was so morose and dark for such a young man. As for Sharon, it wasn't as obvious. I explained to them both what the situation was. We set up a time to meet at the office to do their removals. (These are described in Chapter 4.)

Looking back I'm thinking Taylor knew about the *Attachments* and that drawing us there to move him was part of the bigger purpose of clearing the area of ghosts that could *Attach* to his family in the future.

Taylor is not the only one Robert has encountered that did not transition immediately after death. There are others. Many, many of them. "Sometimes, the ghosts themselves find me.", says Robert. "For instance, one evening while at home on the computer my attention was drawn to the glass half full of water to my right. I saw the glass tip (on its own) to the side just to the point the water was about to spill out. Then, the glass righted itself. I knew straight away someone was on the other side and needed to communicate. So, I met with the appropriate member of my team to communicate with the spirit. It turns out it was the ghost of a man. He was a local policeman who had very recently been shot and killed. He had a message for his wife. I wrote it up and sent it to the family. Afterwards, he was able to move on from his ghosting state to his next place in the afterlife."

Ghosts and *Attachments* have methods of functioning that make them distinct from one another. Not all ghosts *Attach*. Some merely ghost indefinitely. They may be deceased relatives that want to dispense advice or check on their families to see that they are ok. Others may just feel lonely and desire companionship or they may be drawn to places that are familiar to them. Some just like being around the living; others may be drawn to simply interact with the living in non-intrusive ways. For instance, several years ago, during a visit to a Ghost Town in the San Diego area, the Ghost Removers discovered that the ghosts were having fun and enjoying the attention from the visitors in a completely harmless way.

On the other hand some ghosts may want to pressure, manipulate or even control a living person. They may make many attempts before someone responds to them. Once they find a vulnerable human host, they may target that person as a good candidate to *Attach*. Recognizing a weakness in the Subtle Body, they seize the opportunity to initiate a parasitic type relationship.

When ghosts influence, *Attach,* and even possess a person, they are using the only abilities they have at their disposal. Like any ability, when not used properly, it can become potentially harmful, even unintentionally. Even 'good'

186

intentions can have 'bad' consequences.

When examining the Ghost Remover case files for an *Attachment* cycle, it is important to observe the same severity progression regarding the tactics employed by the *Attachment*. As a result, it will become clear that the issue is mostly the result of a succession of events. *Attachment* cases that have increased in severity have some type of progressive change that accompanies the process of an *Attachment* entrenching itself in more firmly. It begins with observing and intelligence gathering. It eventually leads to pressuring and manipulating. And at times it concludes with controlling or possessing a person. In some case, they take-over completely.

Because *Attachment* scenarios can be rooted in haunting, whenever possible, Robert prefers to meet with clients in their own environments. Robert is always careful to be very vigilant when on location for the safety of all involved. Some astonishing things have happened and no session is ever ordinary. The Ghost Remover's stories combined with their client histories are each fascinating in their own way. The more they share these stories in places like ghostremover.com, in local appearances at metaphysical gatherings or on the air on Darkness Radio, the more people haunted by similar afflictions find them for help. After each guest appearance Robert is inundated with queries. Hundreds of people send their information to be checked for the presence of an *Attachment*. Because these people already experience symptoms, *Attachment* rates tend to be higher than average. Some of those people travel from different parts of the country to San Diego for a clearing.

CASE FILE: When it Comes to the Paranormal, Expect the Unexpected

In the following case, the clients were from San Diego so the clearing for them could be done on location. Included here are excerpts from their initial email message to Robert, then what they discovered during the intervention, and that is followed up by their letter back to radio talk show host Dave at Darkness Radio.

> Dear Mr. Major;
>
> Thank you for the enjoyable and enlightening information shared recently on Darkness Radio. We are hopeful that you are the blessing we have been waiting for. Two of us are writing this email to you, Daniela and myself, Susan. As neighbors we live one block from each other and have both had uncomfortable experiences which we strongly feel are paranormal activity in and around our homes.
>
> Activity has gone on now for ten years in my home, I have initially sought the help of the Catholic Church and even went through a Native American cleansing ceremony which brought only temporary relief. Daniela for the first time got proactive and used Holy Water yesterday. She did a blessing after her young daughter saw a shadow presence yesterday morning, but her older daughter still experienced a bad nightmare last night. Neither daughter knew of the other's experience.
>
> Paranormal activity has ranged as follows;
>
> • seeing shadow people in both our homes, the most

recent a week ago in my home and yesterday morning Daniela's 19 year-old daughter witnessed a shadow person dart past the open bathroom door while looking in the mirror while applying make-up.

- objects disappearing.
- violent nightmares that wake me up in a rage and a sweat.
- Daniela's 22 year-old daughter has had violent nightmares since age four or five. Last night she had a nightmare so violent she could not talk about it this morning.
- personal physical attacks, one that caused me to break my wrist, another that catapulted me into an empty Jacuzzi.
- doors slamming, doors being unlocked and opening.

... and more that might be easier to discuss with you directly. May we speak with you? We live in the community of Tierrasanta and are willing to follow your lead. Daniela and I do not feel safe in our homes, especially alone and at night. We are determined, and we refuse to give up. We are grateful for your consideration in this matter.

Bless you and all you do,
Daniella

Robert's response to Daniela went to Susan first because Daniela was having issues with her computer.

...After checking everyone in both houses for

Attachments. You are all *Attached.* Are you available at home this Sunday at noon? I would like to come by with my team to determine the extent of paranormal activity at your homes?

Daniela emailed back,

Dear Robert,

God bless you and thank you for your quick confirmation that we have *Attachments.* This, of course makes me very frightened but also relieved to know that it may be the basis of conflict in our home. My concern is for my daughters.

I called my husband at work today and pretty much begged him to participate. (If you recall, Susan mentioned to you that my husband is neither a supporter nor a believer, and a very devout Catholic.) Susan and I had hoped to do this while he was out of town on the weekend of July 20th or 21st; and we had intended to send the girls away to not cause them any alarm. However, given that he and the girls have *Attachments,* I believe it is important for them to be present. My younger daughter is going out of town tonight, but will be back Saturday. So, this is indeed the weekend all will be here.

May I please have until tomorrow to let you know about this weekend? I would like an opportunity to try to convince my husband as he believes all this is nonsense. I am also concerned about being able to convince my daughters as their fear is giving more power to negativity. They don't even want to talk about it as they are the ones with the experiences. I honestly do not even know how to begin to approach this with my daughters as my younger daughter is going out of town tonight. She will be back Saturday, though. I will have to come up with something, however, as I really do fear for them. I am open to and grateful for any suggestions you may have, Robert.

Susan will be available either weekend. For me, the sooner, the better. I will contact you tomorrow morning if that is ok. Thank you, Robert; and if you cannot wait and must give the Sunday noon appointment to someone else, I do understand. Susan and I thank you with all our hearts. You cannot even imagine what is going through my mind right now. Knowledge is power; though, and I live by that.

Sincerely,
Daniela

Robert recounts what happened next.

"We proceeded to set our intervention for the coming Sunday. *Attachments* can start acting up once they know we are coming after them so we try to get on it right away. I call the team to make sure everyone can make it on Sunday. We have been developing some strong new talent and I wanted them all there to participate for this one."

"The team arrives at noon that Sunday to a

seemingly nice little quaint community. Most houses are tract homes that were built in the 1980's. From the outside everything looks normal but once we walked into Susan's home we could sense the ghostly presence. Today would be special because all the newest members of the team were going to be there. Besides Ghost Remover Brittany, (Charles's granddaughter from a previous Case File) we also had Angelica (associated with one of the Case Files that took place during the 'Sizzle' taping for the Los Angeles production company). Then there is Brett and he ghost hunts using special electronic equipment. He travelled from Los Angeles to sit in on this session. He wanted to test and see if we would be able to collaborate together. We all introduced ourselves and sat for a little bit getting to know one another and learning the history of the house."

"Susan seems so grateful that we are there. She told us she had tried everything possible to no avail. I assured her we would take care of business and not to worry. The team is ready. I have everyone except Brett enter trance and tell them to let me know what they see. They let me know there are numerous ghosts there and they are very angry that we are present. Mostly Native Americans they say, from local area tribes that passed a long time ago. They were buried there and that is why there were so many. Two young children were ghosting and running amok through the home. The first thing we want to do is remove the *Attachments* then we will get to those that are just ghosting."

"A history of both women's *Attachments* is revealed. How they got on, how long they have been on and what they are doing to them. Daniela's *Attachment* was quite angry. Antoinette was telling how the *Attachment* was wagging her finger back and forth as if we were doing something wrong there. That happens sometimes. Antoinette details when the *Attachment* got on. It was in Hawaii around fourteen years ago. Daniela answers that indeed she had travelled to Hawaii during that time. Antoinette says her *Attachment* was carrying a Bible with her so maybe she was a missionary. There are three others also present but do not influence like this one does. They cause physical problems as well they say."

Robert and his team went on to clear the others of their *Attachments*. And then they cleared the area of ghosts. Brett's ghost detecting equipment did not appear to have the frequency and range to pick up on the paranormal activity that day. And, Daniela was so pleased with the clearing, she sent the following letter to Dave at Darkness Radio:

Dear Dave,

First of all, thank you for Darkness Radio. I listen to you and Tim on podcast every day on my walks here in San Diego. I guess you can say you are my 'walking' buddies. Because I listen to you all the time, I know how serious you both are about having credible guests on your show. …That is why I contacted Robert Major without hesitation; and he and his team, (who we have affectionately dubbed "the power rangers"), did not disappoint.

My friend, Susan, had been having disturbing paranormal activity in her home and personal attacks for many years. From apparitions to doors slamming in the middle of the day or night to her being catapulted into her empty Jacuzzi, the list is as long as my forearm. (Susan was a victim of an Apache curse).

Since the day I met her almost a year ago, I was on a quest to help her. We tried many avenues, but to no avail. And then . . . I heard Robert's story. It made sense to me. As I was listening to him speak, I thought "I wonder where he lives and if he would be willing to travel to Susan's home"; and then he said he lived in San Diego. WE CONTACTED HIM IMMEDIATELY.

Robert Major and his power ranger team is wonderful, Dave! From the moment we contacted him, he and his team were right on it. Yes, there were *Attachments,* and last Sunday, Robert and his incredible power rangers removed seven *Attachments* from Susan and six other ghosts from her home. For the first time in many years, Susan slept through the night. Indeed, for the past three nights (since the removals) she has had uninterrupted sleep. She never used to be able to sleep at night. Something would always wake her at 3 am or 4 am without fail and often times with violent nightmares. So, this is a big deal that Susan is able to get a good night's rest. It appears even her cat, Izzy, has benefited. Robert's sister (Antoinette) communicated with Izzy's spirit guide and correctly diagnosed a serious health condition Izzy suffers from. Robert's sister did this without meeting Izzy face to face as the cat was upstairs. Another plus, now Izzy sleeps in her cat bed, something Izzy has not been willing to do for the past two years. She would leap out of it, the minute Susan would put her in it.

Robert is now working with me. He has removed my *Attachments*; but some of my loved ones have *Attachments* as well. Robert and I are hoping to be able to work with my priest to help them. It is not easy, sometimes, when the victims of these *Attachments* are not willing. Susan and I are meeting with my priest tomorrow. I feel it is important for her to be there so she can testify to the positive changes she has experienced in her life. Please keep us in your prayers that we will have my priest's support as this is important to the persons who are *Attached*.

From what I have witnessed, I can see that Robert and his wonderful team of dedicated souls (on this side and the other) are willing to do whatever it takes to rid this world of this terrible and sometimes covert evil. I will be honest and say that I don't know what they do or how they do it; but they certainly get the job done. Maybe, you can have Robert on the show again. I'd really love for you to talk to him about that in greater detail. I think it's important to get this information out there. I still can't believe he was here in San Diego all the time.

In closing, Dave, know that you and Tim and your show really do make a difference. Just think how many lives you have improved with just this one. I always look forward to your podcasts. Maybe, three hours some day? I know, I know, we only recently were granted two hours. We can hope.

God bless you, your work, and your family,
Daniela

A year after the clearing, Susan contacted Robert to say that she was sensing spirit presences about the house again. Robert scheduled to come to Susan's home the following weekend with Ghost Remover Marcos. Marcos cleared the area of some ghosts that were ready to make the transition. Susan asked that her newest roommate be checked for *Attachments*. She had scheduled the appointment for a time he was sure to be at home. After checking, he was indeed *Attached*. However, when Susan went to his room to broach the subject with him to see if he would consider being cleared she found his room vacant and realized that he had slipped out of the house unnoticed down the side entrance. She looked about the room and discovered that he had dark magic paraphernalia in his room that would bring spirits to her home. Upon making the finding, Susan decided it was time to give this new roommate notice to find another place to live so that he would not summon more spirits to her home.

While the Ghost Remover team has been working on location, they've encountered sudden nearby disruptions, outbursts, and even violent confrontations coming from neighboring areas.

CASE FILE: In a Lakeside Trailer Park

Here is what happened.

On one occasion while on location, the Ghost Removers were clearing a family of *Attachments* that resided in a trailer park in Lakeside, CA. Robert realized that *Attachments* on a couple in the adjacent trailer were beginning to act out violently. It is not uncommon for ghosts in the vicinity to act out in response to Ghost Remover team activity. In this case, ghosts *Attached* to the neighbor couple reacted to the removal of ghosts on the clients because it was occurring on a level they could perceive. They were not happy about the removal.

In response to the couple's heated arguments, angry shouts and physical blows, other neighbors phoned 911. Within minutes the police arrived to stop the violent altercation. There was nothing the Ghost Remover team could do in this instance to help the neighboring couple. Therefore, they finished their clearing of the family that had requested their services and left.

Robert is always careful to be vigilant when on location for the safety of all involved. Astonishing things can and do happen.

CHAPTER 13:
THE POLTERGEIST

In cases people sometimes wonder why the Ghost Remover's don't get even more information about the ghosts in the area or *Attachments*. In response, they explain that all of their attention needs to be focused on the removal of these spirits. Once these entities are aware of their abilities to remove and clear them, they can act out. There is often little opportunity to ask more about them. Most of the information they do get comes directly from their Spirit Guides who provides information more on a need to know basis than for curiosity sake. Consequently, some of the Case Files may sound unfinished. Usually, at the conclusion of a removal session, everyone is so relieved it's over, it is only later that they think of questions that they wish they had asked.

Additionally, there is a significant difference between sessions held at the office versus those done on location. The sessions held at the office proceed like this:
- The client is placed in a light hypnotic trance.
- The Ghost Remover is placed in a trance.
- Spirit Guides notified in advance of the appointment are already present and they either assist or possess the team member to work with or through the team member to remove the *Attachment*.

- Through the Spirit Guides, the Ghost Remover often gets essential information about the *Attachment* and relays that information to the client. For instance, how many *Attachments* there are and where in the body they are located. They assess what the *Attachments* are like including personality traits, intention and severity. It is essential to arm themselves with as much information as they can because when they go to remove them, *Attachments* rarely go willingly. Information gleaned during the removal session include some or all of the following:
  - ➢ *Who* the *Attachment(s)* was when alive.
  - ➢ What the client did that attracted the *Attachment(s)* to him in the first place.
  - ➢ Where the client was when he got *Attached*.
  - ➢ Why the client got *Attached*.
  - ➢ The physical, mental or emotional trauma that created the opening the person's subtle body.

The extent some or all of the information is obtained depends upon what transpires during the removal. In some cases it can be like witnessing an abrupt outburst in a crowded bar. Removing the disrupters is much like a bouncer in a bar grabbing an unruly patron and physically throwing him out of an establishment and off the premises. He may even profess his innocence and desire to remain. During these dramatic and intense situations, it is not likely that you could get answers to questions like, who is that, why is he here, what happened or where did he come from. And because it happens so fast, witness accounts may be sketchy. Everyone in the vicinity knows something drastic just happened, but they may not have all the details or facts.

Spirit Guides work with and sometimes through ("possess") the team members. Because the Spirit Guides are on the same 'spiritual realm level' as the *Attachment(s)*, they are able to grab them and take them off the client. *Attachments* often act out just prior to removal trying to attack the team or body-hop. So everyone involved works quickly, kind of like the bouncer in the bar evicting an unruly patron from the premises, just not physically because it occurs on a non-physical level. Together, they remove the *Attachment* and send it on with its own Spirit Guide or Guardian Angel to its next phase of transition. The Ghost Remover team makes no judgment about where that is or why.

Once the *Attachment(s)* are gone, a Ghost Remover team member seals the opening on the Subtle Body that allowed the *Attachment* to enter in the first place. Then communications take place on behalf of the client for any spirit related guidance that can be conveyed to the client. Most guidance is unique to that individual. Typically a client may hear things regarding life issues, health and behavior especially as it relates to how to avoid getting *Attached* in the future. That guidance is often summarized with the statement that: It is up to them to make the necessary adaptations in their lives to avoid becoming *Attached* again.

At that point the human host victim is completely free of the *Attachment(s)* and the Ghost Remover's job is done.

If clients get re-*Attached* in the future, Ghost Removers will clear them. However, if clients get re-*Attached* multiple times and do not make any effort to adjust their behavior which would reduce their susceptibility to *Attachments*, it becomes fruitless and the Ghost Remover team may respectfully decline to continue to clear them until they make the necessary life changes to stop the *Attachment* cycle.

It is possible to verify changes in the Subtle Body and thereby the Ghost Remover process by having a Kirlian or 'aura' photograph taken before and after a removal session. Some clients like to have some kind of verification and are thrilled to be able to see the differences in their before and after 'aura' scans.

Robert always follows up with clients in the weeks following a removal. Very often they say they are experiencing a new sense of clarity and well-being. Many express deep gratitude because they feel they have control over their lives again.

Although most sessions are conducted in their office, sometimes the Ghost Removers work on location. Normally, if on location, the Ghost Remover team will start a session with an assessment process. Is the area haunted? How many ghosts are there? Are any of the people present there *Attached* ? It is important that they identify who is *Attached* as well as what ghosts are in the vicinity. Animals, especially pets are a great source of information on the local ghosts and *Attachments* because they perceive them. The team member that communicates with animals gets as much information from them as possible to help paint a more complete picture of what they are facing. They need to know what they are dealing with before they open a channel.

The Ghost Removers have become highly skilled at

removals. Even with all of their preparation, they know to be on guard for the unexpected. Experience has shown them that *Attachments* can jump (aka body-hop) to another person or even attack team members. If not properly contained, they can even act out through their host. As team leader, Robert maintains control of the session and addresses issues as they arise. Likewise, it is fascinating work because they never know what to expect once they engage the spirit realm. They always walk away with an expanded view of reality and our place within it.

In this next segment, we take a look at the traumatic circumstances surrounding the death of young woman who then became a poltergeist. A poltergeist is a type of ghost capable of interfering with the physical world. In other words, they can, to some extent, transverse realms between ghosting and physical worlds. They are responsible for physical disturbances, such as loud noises and objects being moved or destroyed. They are purportedly capable of striking out at as well as tripping people. As shown in this next case, poltergeist behavior can disrupt living people.

CASE FILE: The Address was "666..."
The following is a summary of Robert's account of what occurred on October 28, 2017.

What we find is that when horrific acts befall a person it just doesn't stop with their death. The ramifications can go on for years and years after the act even into a future life. Therefore, most ghosts we encounter have a sad story to tell. We do our best to change things around for them.

I became introduced to the scenario through a phone call from Angelica. Angelica is our ghost remover team's aura sealer. Her function is to repair openings in the subtle body thereby preventing ghosts from *Attaching* to a living person in the future.

Angelica's cousin Adam was acquainted with her team role. So, when the paranormal activity that had begun a few months prior had escalated to an intolerable level, he called her to tell his story. Adam explained that strange things had been happening in his home for months. He described the paranormal activity as ranging from weird noises in the middle of the night to doors and cabinets were opening and closing on their own. That sort of thing bothered him. But what happened next scared him and his family members. He didn't realize things between a ghost and the living could become physical.

Adam's son was about twenty years old at the time and was living at home at the time. His girlfriend Ellen was staying there too. One night, while alone in her bedroom, Ellen felt herself being attacked by something or someone that she could not see. She screamed out in pain. Adam and his son rushed into the bedroom to investigate. They found Ellen in a state of panic. She was terrified. It might have been possible to discount her account of what happened except when examining Ellen's back under her shirt they found deep scratches. One ran the entire length of her spine. They took photos of the scratches.

After hearing Adam's story and seeing the photos, Angelica called me. We set an appointment for the coming Saturday midday. I always feel more confident doing our work during the daylight hours. Team members are more alert during the day. This is important because we all need to be hyper-vigilent once we enter a scene. In addition to being observant in the physical world, we watch out for each other for anything coming our way in the spirit realms.

I was taken aback when Angelica conveyed the street address to me. The first three numbers were 666. I do not equate these numbers with the devil, but some do. So, I couldn't help but notice the coincidence between the interpretations some of have the numbers and the activity happening at the house.

Next, I contact Ghost Remover Antoinette who in turn notifies the appropriate spirit guides that their assistance will also be required during the appointment. The ghosts we encounter in the office during *Attachment* removals is often of a different nature than when going out on location. When on location, we never know what scenario we are walking into because time does not exist in the ghost realm. Therefore we find spirits of the dead existing in the same places as the living. Once we open up a channel into these other realms, the situation can unravel fast. Given the nature of the paranormal activity Adam described, I phone Marcos and ask that he attend the appointment as well.

Once the appointment is made, very often the offending ghost(s) and even ghosts in the area will begin to act out because, like the proverbial fly-on-the-wall relationship, they are aware of what the client's intentions for the appointment are.

The appointment is not designed to meet and get to know the ghost as in getting to know a guest staying at the home of a friend. Instead, it is orchestrated to remove the ghost who has invaded the client and/or their property. Then, to pass it on to its spirit guide who handles it from there. As a result, energetically strong and highly emotional ghosts do all they can to influence, disrupt or even possess the client in an effort to insure the appointment does not take place. Sometimes they are successful, other times not.

There are many factors involved such as:
- The prospective client's belief system; i.e.: religion etc.
- Social pressures.
- Strength and influence of the ghost(s).
- Whether or not the residents of the home have fallen victims to the point of being *Attached* or even possessed by one or more spirits of the dead. In these cases, we clear the person as well as the property.

I arrived at the house on the appointed day. The home is situated in an older part of San Diego in an established neighborhood built during the 1950s. Once I google searched the address. Upon seeing the map of the area, I recognized the area straight away as being one I was familiar with. Whether passing through it or as a destination, it felt to me as if it had a dark cloud over it. Some people would describe it as having 'bad energy'. While traveling past an invisible boundary of this half mile section of town I experience the feeling as if a dark cloud suddenly passed and the sun's rays burst through. The surrounding area feels bright and shiny.

The homes on the street consist of larger 1800 square feet

ranch style homes on ¼ to ½ acre lots. Paint is faded. Devoid of lawns, there is dirt. They are not unkempt. Instead they were all simply at the same stage of aging. The paint on all of them appeared to have faded in the harsh desert-like sun at the same rate.

Antoinette had arrived at the same time as myself for our twelve o'clock appointment. It was a mild temperature sunny southern California day. After exiting my vehicle, entering the area on foot felt more like what I'd imagine first responders coming upon a violent crime scene. There was mayhem. We walked up to Angelica who was with a group of people gathered around an SUV that was parked in the double wide driveway. Everyone one was talking at the same time. Their agitation carried by the breeze from the sound of their voices met my ears. My eyes picked up on the fear in their facial expressions.

Angelica introduced myself and Antoinette to Adam and the others gathered there. Adam was the first to give his account of the paranormal activity that Angelica had already conveyed to me during the intake and appointment setting phone call.

His car keys were in one hand. His cell phone in the other. "Look" Adam said while pointing to the picture on his cell phone of the scratches on his son's girlfriend's back. Expanding the image view, their presence became clearer. I could see patches of scratches. The full back length one however, was deeper than a scratch and more like a gouge. That must have hurt.

A ghost who inflicts physical damage is referred to as a poltergeist. In this case, the ghost scratched the gal. In other cases we have found that they can disrupt technology, throw objects, cause things to fall from overhead, and in one instance, operate a driverless vehicle. In one such case, I was injured a few years ago when a poltergeist abruptly unhinged a several hundred pound Murphy bed from the wall causing it to fall and hit me in the back of my head and upper back. Needless to say I am extra careful these days.

Adam's son and girlfriend were clearly upset. She had no idea how this could have happened to her. While he was concerned for her safety and well being.

It was apparent that *everyone* in that group was scared! They'd all experienced some paranormal activity at the house during the past few months. They remained on the property only long enough after we arrived to give their authorization for us to enter and clear the premises. Telling me that they would return in a few hours, then, they separated in several groups, loaded themselves up in the SUV and another vehicle and sped away. We were left to deal with the problem on our own.

Marcos was on his way from his day job. Things must have occurred that delayed him because he was late to the appointment.

In the meantime, Angelica, Antoinette, Robert and L. Sims were gathered in the chairs that were situated in the large shaded foyer between the garage and the home.

We know ghosts can act out and felt confident, given the description of the paranormal activity described by Adam and his family that this ghost already was aware of our presence. In anticipation of Marcos' imminent arrival, I placed Antoinette in trance so that spirit guide Lane could speak to me directly through her without the need for interpretation.

Through the Spirit Guides, the Ghost Remover often gets essential information about the ghost(s) whenever possible. For instance, how many there are and where they are located. They assess these spirits of the dead for personality traits, intention and severity. It is essential to arm themselves with as much information as they can because when they go on location to remove them, ghost(s) rarely go willingly.

In cases where Antoinette is interpreting for a spirit entity she will use references to "S/he said." However, when possessed by an entity, the spirit will speak in the first person and use the term "I". In this instance, Antoinette's spirit was not in possession of her body and I was speaking directly with a spirit guide named Lane. Lane is our go-to guide for working with ghosting spirits of the dead.

Lane could sense the strength of this ghost and did not want to engage it in advance of everyone on the team being present and ready to set foot in the house. While waiting, we made small chat. The entrance to the house from the foyer was secured by two doors. The security door was closed in place in front of the wooden door that was also in a closed position behind it. All of a sudden, as if some invisible person burst out of the house, the security door flung open and banged loudly as it slammed into the side of the house.

Everyone on the team is used to such occurrences. They do

not frighten us. However, they provide clues into the characteristics about the ghosts we need to know about.

Marcos arrived. We apprised him of the situation and the security door flinging open. From experience, we all know to be on high alert. We entered the house from the foyer through the long galley style kitchen to the dining area. Upon entering I quickly scan for knives and other dangerous implements that could be thrown our way. There were none.

I have Antoinette and Marcos take a seat at the round wooden kitchen table which was surrounded by four matching chairs. Antoinette faced the opening to the living room. Marcos faced the kitchen we had just entered from. For Marcos, the living room was to his left.

Antoinette was still in trance. Spirit guide Lane was within contact range. We could feel the presence in the house and I wanted to get right to work so it couldn't escape. I placed Marcos in trance. He is a remote viewer and can perceive the scene from other points of view outside of the range of physical senses. He saw the ghost sitting in the living room chair. He described her vitality as strong. Her demeanor was angry.

Antoinette can also see ghosts while in trance. Both Antoinette and spirit guide Lane identify one ghost on the premises. They motion towards the living room saying they see the ghost of a young woman sitting in the recliner. They describe her as having a defiant look.

Armed with the knowledge that they had only one ghost to deal with, they proceeded with caution. The ghost remember team members both here and in the spirit realm work together to corral the ghost so that she cannot escape.

Suddenly, Marcos shouts out "Shut up" as a means of relaying to us what the ghost is saying. Marcos translates more for us. She's saying that she doesn't like the gal she scratched (Ellen) at all. That is why she attacked her.

The ghost communicates through Marcos that she has been present in this area since the Great Depression. She was only sixteen when she was murdered in 1936. She stated that she knew the murderer but he was never caught. She says that the belief held just after the murder was that she had been killed by the someone described in modern terms as a serial killer. She did not use that term but meant the same thing so we'll use that term here.

She said she was so angry that her life had been taken from her at such a young age. As a result, she didn't care for anyone or anything. Ghosts were people too. We are empathetic for what they experienced in life and compassion for the unfortunate state we find them in as a ghost. Each story is unique but their predicaments have the same common elements.

By allowing her the freedom to express, Marcos has attracted her to enter the kitchen like a bee to a flower. Once close enough, he grabs her. He has her in his grasp as any bouncer would have an unruly patron he must eradicate from a bar. She fights back but is contained by a type of force field he has created.

Ghosts consider transition a kind of death. Because they didn't transition to the afterlife at death they are afraid of moving on. They therefore see it as the death they never had to experience. But in fact, their spirit guides are waiting for them as they have been all along to help them transition."

This ghost is handed over to the spirit guides who have been waiting there for her all along to transition. By aiding in her transition from here to the afterlife she can finally find peace and move forward.

Information gleamed at the time of the removal can be sketchy. When the opportunity presents itself, we inquire as to:

➤ *Who* the *Attachment(s)* was when alive.
➤ What the client did that attracted the *Attachment(s)* to him in the first place.
➤ Where the client was when he got *Attached.*
➤ Why the client got *Attached.*
➤ The physical, mental or emotional trauma that created the opening the person's subtle body.

People sometimes wonder why the Ghost Remover's don't get even more information about the ghost(s). In response, we explain that all of our attention needs to be focused on the ghost removal. Once these entities are aware of their abilities to remove and clear them, they can act out. There is often little opportunity to ask more about them.

Most of the information we do get comes directly from their Spirit Guides who provides information more on a need to know basis than for curiosity sake. Consequently, some of the Case Files may sound unfinished. Usually, at the conclusion of a removal session, everyone is so relieved it's over, it is only later that we think of questions that we wished we had asked.

In this case, we check with spirit guide Lane for any additional information he might have that could shed light on what occurred or who she was. He did not.

Sometimes more information is forthcoming if we ask to be updated by the spirit guides in attendance. Since we made the inquiry, he agreed to check in with the spirit guides who are with the ghost for an update.

Afterwards, the whole house felt lighter. Adam and his family report that they have not experienced any further paranormal activity in their home. They express profuse gratitude. And, once I apprised them of the ghost's history, they have a new appreciation for what she experienced along with a sense of compassion for ghosts in general.

Three days afterwards, Lane (through Antoinette) provides me with an update on our Ghost. He told us that her spirit guides were helping her through the grieving process of what happened to her bringing her life to such an abrupt and dreadful end. We learn she is making slow progress and they anticipate it will take her some time to work through the trauma. They gave us her name. Celia Cota.

Robert followed up by performing in internet search for Celia Cota. Information in articles printed about Celia's case coincided with what Robert and his team learned during this case.

First, the Madera Tribune article entitled *Seventh Fiend Crime San Diego Discovered Young Girl is Victim* dated August 18, 1934 which described the events surrounding Celia Cota's demise.

The following is a picture of Celia published at the time of her death.

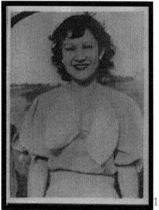

14

Secondly, in an article entitled *Sex Crimes Are Studied By Officers* published in the Madera Tribune, Number 270, 17, January, 1947 compares the brutal murders of Celia Cota and seven other unsolved murders, one of which was that of Celia Cota.

The tragic story of Celia Cota who had her life shortened in a horrific way became the type of ghost known as a poltergeist. She had the ability to move objects like slamming open the security door and cause other disruptions in the residence. She also used her capabilities to harm a living person by severely scratching a woman's back. This behavior can appear demon-like.

---

14 Photos Source Unknown.

However, in Celia's case, she was not a demon. Instead, she was traumatized and therefore an angry spirit of the dead with poltergeist capabilities. By associating her name with a picture of her face and description of her poltergeist behavior it is can become clearer that *ghosts of living human beings, were at one time, people too!*

There are many kinds of emotional trauma. Being the victim of a crime is certainly one of the worst traumas one could experience. Ghost Remover case files are full of physically and emotionally traumatized people who have come to them for *Attachment* removals. Quite often, the ghost has their own traumatic story too.

The Ghost Remover team includes a core group of spirit guides and helpers. One specifically has the role of identifying whether or not a prospective client is *Attached*. Some guide the clearing process. Others function as Spirit Operators who enter into and possess a Ghost Remover Channel so that they can work from the Subtle Body and Spirit Body levels *into* the physical world. In this way, Ghost Removers work from the physical *into* the non-physical realms. In the end, Spirit helpers hand off the wayward, sometimes traumatized, spirits to the spirit guide that has been waiting all along to help them move on to the afterlife.

No Ghost Remover session is ever ordinary. These stories combined with client histories are each fascinating in their own way.

You may even begin to recognize that some of these behaviors are familiar to you. In fact, we have all interacted with someone who is *Attached* but just weren't aware of it. After becoming familiar with the signs, you will be able to see it for yourself.

CHAPTER 14:
GHOST REMOVER PROCESS
AND BEYOND

The Ghost Remover process has come a long way from the first removal which took place around the year 2000 when during a session, Hypnotherapist Robert Major stumbled upon an *Attachment* situation and became aware of its implications for the *Attached* person. During that session, Robert was spirit guided to help the client with an *Attachment* removal. The entire process took about an hour. Unlike most spiritual communicators, the Ghost Remover team is unique in its incorporation of trance and spirit guides to deal with these entities that have been disrupting people's lives. In summary, *Attachments* are working from the spirit realm to the physical. Ghost Removers are working from the physical to the spirit realm. The process continues to shift and evolve as their skills refine, new members join the team and different client situations present them with new challenges.

Since the time of that first removal, Robert carefully moved forward to assemble a team. Interestingly, of the many people who have found their way to Robert for help, some have been identified by the Ghost Remover team's spirit guides who, from their vantage point, are easily able to identify those with remarkable abilities that can help the team. They communicate that information to Robert. Some of those talented people have joined the group. Each new team member has the heightened sensitivity to perceiving *Attachments* themselves along with other talents. Their diverse abilities coupled with trance work expand the ordinary to extraordinary.

They use a team approach to insure that the necessary skill-sets for the task at hand are readily available because things can happen fast and they want to be well prepared. It is important that nothing gets missed or overlooked. Over time, they cross-train on different specialties.

They are also unique in their use of trance state to access these invisible dimensions. Trance work is the technique by which they fine tune their access to a channel which functions like an opening or portal. The portal the dark spirits use to enter our world is the path the Ghost Remover team members follow while in trance to get into their realm. They have spirit guides who protect them when accessing these realms. Conversely, these helping spirits have chosen Ghost Remover team members as their conduit to the living. The Ghost Remover team could not know what the *Attachments* are doing if they were unable to traverse these realms safely.

Robert acts as a guide for his team. During sessions he anchors Ghost Remover team members in this world and guides them back into their bodies when the sessions conclude. It is this process that makes exploring the invisible spirit realms possible.

The Spirit Guides who work with the Ghost Remover team from the spirit realm have areas of specialties as well and are called upon to help out when their particular expertise are required. They consist of spirits all operating on different levels with different frequencies or ranges. Think of the spirit realms as a sort of school. Some are at lower frequencies which would make them closer in range to the physical world of the living. These are the guides and teachers providing help for the 'students', still others, whose frequency is even higher are the teachers of the teachers and so on.

Currently, there about a dozen spirit guides they work with on a regular basis. They have developed an additional network of contacts in the spirit realm to reach the particular Spirit Guide who is needed at any given time. As a result, the Ghost Remover team of spirit guides and metaphysically gifted helpers that have been carefully assembled over time have become highly effective.

The Ghost Remover teams of spirit guides and metaphysically gifted helpers that have been carefully assembled over time have become highly effective. The Ghost Remover team has developed long term relationships with spirit helpers whose job it is to help these wayward spirits that ghost and *Attach* move on to the appropriate spirit realm they were originally destined for. These Spirit guides chose to establish this relationship with the Ghost Removers as their conduit to the living. They are purely interested in helping these lost spirits find their way and have guided Robert and his team from the start. The spirit helpers and having pure intentions are essential to the team's success.

The Ghost Remover process begins with an *Attachment* assessment. When a potential client contacts Robert, he asks them to provide their birth date and full name at birth. Although this data may seem serendipitous, it is actually very fundamentally significant information. Very much like the GPS (Global Positioning Satellite) device on your cell phone that can provide its (and therefore your) location no matter where you are, the spirit guides can identify anyone within humankind that has ever lived or is currently living from that data. With that information they can focus in on any person and check to see if he is *Attached*.

In the majority of cases, Robert calls Antoinette once a week where he places her into trance over the phone. Robert transmits the list of names and birthdates to check for that week to her spirit guide(s). The spirit guides are careful to avoid detection so as not to alert or alarm the *Attachments* that an inquiry has been made as to their presence. As a result, the Spirit Guide generally only replies as to whether or not the person in question is or is not *Attached*.

A few days later Robert meets with Antoinette in person. After placing her in trance, she communicates with the spirit guides who have, over the last few days, checked each individual for the presence of an *Attachment*. In other cases, the Spirit Guide comes '*In*' and relays the information personally. After the session is completed, Robert then contacts the client with the status.

Those people that are identified as being *Attached* are invited to come to the San Diego office for a *removal*. Appointments are set. Some fly in from different parts of the country since, based upon Ghost Remover's experience, this process cannot be accomplished successfully on a remote basis.

Once the appointment is made, very often the *Attachments* will begin to act out because, like the proverbial fly-on-the-wall relationship, they are aware of what the client's intentions for the appointment are.

The appointment is not designed to meet and get to know the *Attachment* as in a psychotherapy session. Instead, it is orchestrated to remove the ghost who has invaded the client and pass it on to its spirit guide who handles it from there. As a result, severe *Attachments* do all they can to influence, disrupt or even possess the client in an effort to insure the client does *not* make his appointment. Sometimes they are successful, other times not. There are many factors involved such as:

- The prospective client's belief system; i.e.: religion etc.
- Social pressures.
- Strength and influence of the *Attachment(s)*.
- Who the appointment was scheduled with – the actual person or an *Attachment* that had possessed the individual at the time.

The Ghost Remover team is assembled in preparation for the appointment. Not every team member is needed for each client. From experience and spirit guidance, Robert determines who to include in the session.

Robert Major and the Ghost Remover team hope to bring attention to the *Attachment* epidemic. It is their hope that by exposing the nature of these *Attachments* and the harm they can inflict that they will be able to reach and thereby help a lot more people.

Their goals include expanding their work to include training other teams and traveling to help those who cannot come to them. They endeavor to educate and thereby help not only the people that are *Attached,* but the lost spirits that need to move on from ghosting. Perhaps through their efforts a new understanding of personal distress and dis-ease can provide relief for sufferers that have not been able to find the help they need to live happy and productive lives.

Aspects of what Robert Major has experienced are presented in this book in an effort to share what Robert and his team now understand as a result of their explorations and work. His view of the world and our place within it is forever changed and so are the lives of the people he encounters.

However, their story, like our very nature as human beings is complex. It is much more dimensional than what has been presented here. The main intention here has been to introduce the reader to the topic, which is that living people are interacting with the spirit world all of the time and in different ways. They have spirit guides who are constantly trying to guide them, and they can become enmeshed with wandering earthbound spirits that are no longer alive, but have not moved on to the other realms. These entities disrupt people's lives making their problems harder than they need to be. Robert is dedicated to helping people that have problems arising from these types of entanglements.

Attachments are in fact quite common. By now, it should be evident that *Attachments* are indeed problematic. They plague the living, but to what extent? The only unofficial statistic available is that; on average, one-in-four people who request to be checked for the presence of an *Attachment* through Robert are *Attached*. We can also look to history for confirmation that they exist. There are many references to 'demon possessions' etc. that are now written off as old superstitions that were likely examples of this affliction.

Now you might ask: "What can a person do to reduce the threat of becoming *Attached?*" There is no definitive way to prevent *Attachments* beyond maintaining a healthy lifestyle. While no one is entirely immune, there are steps one can take similar to the guidelines for disease prevention. Living a well-rounded life that includes a healthy diet, exercise, balance, and emotional stability all contribute to a sturdy unflawed Subtle Body which greatly limits intrusions.

Most of the measures center around a healthy lifestyle. If you maintain a strong body and a centered balanced state of mind with good quality social interactions then *Attachments* will have a difficult time exploiting a weakness because there isn't one in regards to way of life. Other tactics to keep in mind to protect oneself are:
- Avoid substance abuse.
- Refrain from unhealthy addictions.
- Avoid situations and places where *Attachments* are prevalent such as the ones mentioned in previous chapters.
- Seek healthy support systems during periods of life

changes and traumatic events.

- Avoid unhealthy thoughts; strive to be positive and optimistic.
- Maintain physical health and a proper diet.

All of these measures can certainly benefit anyone. Beyond being free from past physical, mental and emotional trauma, there are few ways to reduce the probability of *Attachments* getting a foothold on you. That is because the physical, mental and emotional traumas of the general population has resulted in fertile grounds of potential victims which has led to the *Invisible Epidemic* Robert Major describes today. And, the problem is growing each and every day, exponentially, as the population grows.

Because there is no real preventative measure, nor is there a Ghost Remover on every main street as there was a few hundred years ago. Outside of the Ghost Removers, there are few places, if any, to get *Attachments* removed.

So, while taking care of one's own health which in turn strengthens the Subtle Body, that alone unfortunately does not necessarily repair the Subtle Body. And, there are *Attachments* that will seek out a host who has an opening in their aura whether or not they live a clean life. There are *Attachments* that will seek a host who is intoxicated. Other *Attachments* seek out those in pain or even heightened emotions stemming from predicaments of a loved one. As a result, in this day and age, even when in places where one seeks out help, no one is immune from *Attachments* and no place can be considered safe from them.

The Ghost Removers are doing everything they can to

eradicate the problem whenever they encounter it. They hope to spread awareness so that they can help all involved. This includes aiding the spirits lost in transition to locate the source of help they need from their spirit guide who has been waiting for them all along. And, the victims of these lost souls that get *Attached* and even possessed by them.

But when someone gets *Attached*, that is when the Ghost Removers can help. That is not to say that they treat or cure sickness. What personal issues a person had prior to the *Attachment(s)* remain. They only remove *Attachments* and thereby free the victims of their influence. They repair and close the opening in the Subtle Body to keep the person from getting *re-Attached* again in the future. Their goal is to stop the *Attachment* cycle in its tracks. The Ghost Remover team clears victims of these *Attachments* in order to give them unadulterated control over their own lives. Over time they have carefully explored and developed the process that they use today.

IMPORTANT DISCLAIMER

**GHOST REMOVERS DO NOT DIAGNOSE,
TREAT OR CURE ANYTHING.
ATTACHMENTS ARE GHOSTS.
WHAT PERSONAL ISSUES A PERSON HAD PRIOR TO
THE *ATTACHMENT* REMAIN. THEY ONLY REMOVE
ATTACHMENTS AND THEREBY FREE THE VICTIMS
OF THEIR INFLUENCE.**

Epilogue

While researching and writing this book I also uncovered historical facts that trace events which contributed to the mess we in the West find ourselves in today regarding the basis for modern diagnosis and treatment of the *Attached*.

Up Next:
Ghosts, Demons, and Dissociative Identity Disorder: exploring different perspectives to uncover core truths about this multifaceted dilemma.

ABOUT THE AUTHOR

It wasn't until I became personally *Attached* that I came to understand the nature of ghosts that influence, haunt, *Attach* to, and in some cases, take over a human host. When I was cleared of the severe *Attachment* I gained a true appreciation for Robert Major and his Ghost Remover team. That was a big turning point for me.

Prior to that pivotal point, the first two decades of my life after graduating from a Midwestern university in 1980 with a B.S. in Marketing, was spent in the financial services industry sales, marketing and management. In 2001, my path took an abrupt turn and I left the industry. Because that happened, days later, I was present from the first episode forward when Robert Major began exploring the spiritual realm. I have followed Robert Major's hypnosis exploration for nearly twenty years now which has positioned me well to write about it.

Since leaving the financial services industry I earned a certificate from an unaccredited Southern California area Subtle Body Energy School. From there I explored cranial sacral training. I became a licensed minister of the Universal Life Church and began to practice what is best described as Subtle Body Conscious Based Therapy which is a form of Complementary and Alternative Medicine. Since that time I'd undertaken creating a book series on the Subtle Body in regards to wellness and spirituality.

However, as a result of having become *Attached* and subsequently cleared, I put all my attention toward applying what I now know to writing and publishing the book series *Ghost News Source.*

> ➤ *Volume I: The Ghost Remover Chronicles*

> ➤ *Volume II: Ghosts, Demons, and Dissociative Identity Disorder: exploring different perspectives to uncover core truths about this multifaceted dilemma.*

Made in the USA
Columbia, SC
04 August 2019